UNDERSTANDING
PERSON-CENTRED
CARE

for Nursing Associates

Sara Miller McCune founded SAGE Publishing in 1965 to support the dissemination of usable knowledge and educate a global community. SAGE publishes more than 1000 journals and over 800 new books each year, spanning a wide range of subject areas. Our growing selection of library products includes archives, data, case studies and video. SAGE remains majority owned by our founder and after her lifetime will become owned by a charitable trust that secures the company's continued independence.

Los Angeles | London | New Delhi | Singapore | Washington DC | Melbourne

MYLES HARRIS

UNDERSTANDING PERSON-CENTRED CARE

for Nursing Associates

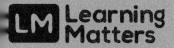
LM Learning Matters

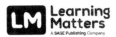

Learning Matters
A SAGE Publishing Company
1 Oliver's Yard
55 City Road
London EC1Y 1SP

SAGE Publications Inc.
2455 Teller Road
Thousand Oaks, California 91320

SAGE Publications India Pvt Ltd
B 1/I 1 Mohan Cooperative Industrial Area
Mathura Road
New Delhi 110 044

SAGE Publications Asia-Pacific Pte Ltd
3 Church Street
#10-04 Samsung Hub
Singapore 049483

Editors: Donna Goddard and Laura Walmsley
Development editor: Eleanor Rivers
Senior project editor: Chris Marke
Marketing manager: George Kimble
Cover design: Wendy Scott
Typeset by: C&M Digitals (P) Ltd, Chennai, India
Printed in the UK

First published in 2021

Library of Congress Control Number: 2020949583

British Library Cataloguing in Publication Data

A catalogue record for this book is available from the British Library

ISBN 978-1-5297-0892-9
ISBN 978-1-5297-0891-2 (pbk)

At SAGE we take sustainability seriously. Most of our products are printed in the UK using responsibly sourced papers and boards. When we print overseas we ensure sustainable papers are used as measured by the PREPS grading system. We undertake an annual audit to monitor our sustainability.

Contents

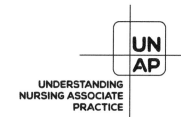

UNDERSTANDING NURSING ASSOCIATE PRACTICE

Supporting you through your nursing associate training & career

UNDERSTANDING NURSING ASSOCIATE PRACTICE is a series uniquely designed for trainee nursing associates.

Each book in the series is:

- Mapped to the NMC standards of proficiency for nursing associates
- Affordable
- Full of practical activities & case studies
- Focused on clearly explaining theory & its application to practice

Current books in the series include:

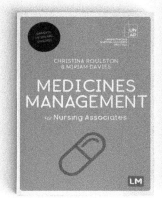

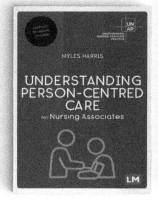

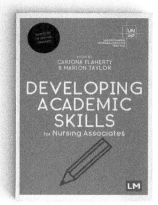

Visit
uk.sagepub.com/UNAP
for more information

About the Author

Myles Harris is an adult nurse and has an MA in practice education. He is a fellow of the Royal Geographical Society, a senior fellow of the Higher Education Academy, and a registered nurse teacher. He worked as a senior lecturer at London South Bank University (LSBU) and was a course director for the FDSc nursing associate apprenticeship. He had a leading role in the team at LSBU, who provided 2 of the 11 test sites for the national development of the nursing associate role. The pilot course at LSBU was shortlisted for nursing associate training programme provider of the year at the Student Nursing Times Awards 2019.

Myles is currently studying for his PhD in risk and disaster reduction at University College London. He is working in collaboration with the not-for-profit organisation Remote Area Risk International and the Royal Centre for Defence Medicine, Ministry of Defence. His research focuses on the education of people providing prolonged field care (healthcare) in remote environments and space.

Acknowledgements

I would like to thank my family and friends, particularly those who are health and social care professionals; you have the highest standards of person-centred care and have provided me with inspiration for the case studies in this book. Thank you to the reviewers of this book, who have provided welcomed challenges and enrichment to the content. A special thank you to the editing team at SAGE, especially Donna Goddard, Laura Walmsley and Ellie Rivers, for their constructive feedback and consistent support throughout many months of writing. Lastly, I would like to thank all of the nursing associates I have taught, whose enthusiasm and hunger to learn inspire me – I wish you all the very best in your lifelong studies and careers.

I dedicate this book to Dr Richard Johnson and Dr Janice Jones. I am very fortunate to know them as colleagues, mentors and friends; their belief in me is invaluable.

Introduction

Who is this book for?

This book has been written primarily for apprentice nursing associates. The content is aimed at addressing the academic and clinical learning needs within your scope of practice. The language used is equally balanced between having strong academic rigour yet remaining accessible. Apprentice nursing associates, however, are not the only audience that will find this book relevant to their practice.

Registered nursing associates who would like to refresh their knowledge of applying theory to practice to achieve person-centred care will find this book useful. Apprentice nursing associates' supervisors, practice development nurses and clinically based education leads will be able to use this book to enhance their understanding of what apprentice nursing associates can do and how they support the provision of evidence-based, person-centred care. Similarly, university academic staff and education providers will find that this book complements their teaching and can be used for blended learning for apprentice nursing associates, as well as an addition to reading lists.

About the book

This book has been written to achieve one aim: introduce holistic, evidence-based and person-centred care to apprentice nursing associates. Achieving this aim will strengthen your sense of professional identity within the multidisciplinary team (MDT) and consolidate your clinical practice in person-centred care. However, this is a complex challenge. As you can see from the table of contents, there is a wide variety of topics covered in this book. This is a reflection of the broad scope of practice that apprentice nursing associates are required to understand and demonstrate.

Nursing associates are generalist practitioners, which makes them unique in the MDT. By the end of your apprenticeship, you will be able to care for people across the lifespan within any field of nursing: adult, paediatric, mental health and learning disability. No other profession has this experience during their training. This book will support you throughout your apprenticeship and during the transition to becoming a registered nursing associate. You should use this book as a springboard that supports your academic studies and enhances your person-centred practice. The chapters have been organised in a progressive structure to enable you to read from beginning to end, or to dip in anywhere if you prefer.

Book structure

Chapter 1, 'Providing person-centred care', is your foundation stone. It provides a brief commentary of the historical events that led to the creation of the nursing associate profession and an overview of the modern NHS system. It identifies how you, once registered as a nursing associate, will fit into the MDT, as well as the unique role you will have. Once the context of nursing associates is established, the key underlying principles of person-centred care are defined. There is an emphasis on developing self-awareness during this chapter, as well as promoting your understanding about how this can affect and benefit patients.

As previously mentioned, one of the factors that makes nursing associates unique is the breadth of their education during the FDSc apprenticeship. Once registered, nursing associates will be able to care for any patients in all clinical environments. Chapter 2, 'Acute and long-term care', reflects the broad scope of practice that apprentice nursing associates need to learn about, providing case studies across the lifespan in all four fields of nursing.

Chapter 3, 'Healthcare ethics and law', introduces the legislation and key documents that underpin professional practice as a nursing associate. Each law and key document are discussed separately, with case studies for each one that exemplify how they apply to clinical practice. The second half of the chapter explores the principles of ethics in healthcare. The content of the chapter examines the philosophies of ethics and encourages nursing associates to debate issues, thinking 'outside the box'. Patient safety and safeguarding are included in the chapter, which are integral responsibilities of nursing associate practice. A common theme throughout the chapter is the provision of person-centred care.

Chapter 4, 'Palliative and end of life care', focuses on caring for patients at the end of their lives (end of life care) and the management of long-term conditions (palliative care). Nursing associates are guided through the knowledge and skills required to meet the needs of dying patients and those living with long-term conditions. There are differences in the care you provide for adults and children at the end of their lives, which are also discussed in this chapter.

A fundamental part of person-centred care is to respect and understand the diversity of the patient population for whom nursing associates will care. Chapter 5, 'Inclusivity in person-centred care', distinguishes the differences between culture, religion and spirituality. There will be suggestions on how reasonable adjustments can be made to accommodate patients' and their families' or friends' diversities during the provision of care. This chapter is in reference to the nine protected characteristics of the Equality Act 2010.

In Chapter 6, 'Public health', it is explained how the social determinants of health support nursing associates in understanding the socio-economic background to patients' health. Furthermore, understanding the local patient population and the community you serve is vitally important to be able to provide person-centred care. With this in mind, this chapter explains how to interpret public health statistics and what they mean for the patients in your care. Obtaining this knowledge and understanding its significance will enable you to provide person-centred care in whichever area of the country you work.

Chapter 7, 'Health promotion and practice education', focuses on how nursing associates can promote the health and wellbeing of the patients in their care, as well as how to provide education when it is appropriate to do so. This broad chapter includes topics such as how to advise patients about a balanced diet, smoking cessation and mindfulness. Moreover, critical thinking skills are developed within the context of critiquing public health campaigns. The importance of a collaborative approach to promoting good physiological and psychological health is emphasised. Patient education is a significant part of the nursing associate role. An objective of this chapter is to build your confidence in patient education by providing a toolkit of techniques that you can apply in practice. Patient education will support nursing associates to be dynamic with their communication, depending on whether they are caring for expert patients or people living with additional learning needs, or conversing with colleagues in the MDT.

Chapter 8, 'Your future in person-centred care', is an innovative chapter on a topic that has not been widely written about. Self-care and the care of your colleagues are integral to ensure that the workforce of a healthcare service is fully functioning to provide person-centred care. This chapter incorporates time management advice on how to enable breaks and the development of coping strategies to lessen the impact of busy, stressful shifts. In addition, this chapter discusses what it means to be a team player and how to support all of your colleagues. This chapter summarises the knowledge and skills learned throughout the book and equips you with the knowledge to maintain continuing professional development (CPD). Finally, there is content on the knowledge and skills needed to keep up to date with the ever-evolving NHS, including new therapies, political influence and technological interventions, while maintaining a person-centred approach to care. The future of health and social care will be dramatically different to recent history, and you will play a valuable role in providing person-centred care.

As a final note on the structure of this book, each chapter has regular subheadings that provide you with a natural break. These are good opportunities for you to pause your study for a short while and then come back to the book feeling refreshed. There are also regular reminders of what has been covered and where the chapter is going next to help you draw together the learning points. Limiting yourself to just reading, however, can only get you so far. Throughout the book, there are a variety of learning features for you to engage with that will support your application of theory to clinical practice.

Requirements for the NMC *Standards of Proficiency for Nursing Associates*

The Nursing and Midwifery Council (NMC) has established standards of proficiency to be met by applicants to different parts of the register, and these are the standards it considers necessary for safe and effective practice. This book is structured so that it will help you to understand and meet the proficiencies required for entry to the NMC register as a nursing associate. The relevant proficiencies are presented at the start of each chapter so that you can clearly see which ones the chapter addresses. The proficiencies have been designed to be generic, so they apply to all fields of nursing and all care settings. This is because all nursing associates must be able to meet the needs of any person they encounter in their practice, regardless of their stage of life or health challenges, whether these are mental, physical, cognitive or behavioural.

This book includes the latest standards for 2018 onwards, taken from the *Standards of Proficiency for Nursing Associates* (NMC, 2018a).

Learning features

Textbooks can be intimidating and learning from reading literature is not always easy. However, this series has been designed specifically for nursing associates. Engaging in the learning features throughout the books will help you to develop your understanding of theory and apply it to practice. This book contains activities, case studies, theory summaries, annotated further reading, and useful websites to enable you to participate in your own learning. The book cannot provide all the answers, but instead provides a good outline of the most important information and helps you to build a framework for your own learning.

It is important to note that for many nursing associates, this apprenticeship will be their first formal education for a long time, or higher education may be a completely new experience. This book aims to support you, presenting theory in an accessible and engaging way. Working in health and social care is an active job that requires the application of practical skills and the use of knowledge and critical thinking skills. The learning features throughout this book complement these requirements and will support you throughout your apprenticeship.

There are a number of activities embedded within each chapter, the aim of which is to enable you to self-assess your learning from the text you have just read. Activities are *not* a test of how well you can memorise things. By completing them, you will develop skills such as critical thinking, reflection, and wider research or reading. Engaging in activities will help you to move the learning points from your short-term memory to long-term memory, and will further enable you to develop the lifelong skills you will need to be able to provide person-centred care as a nursing associate.

Before starting your apprenticeship, you may have worked as a healthcare support worker (HCSW) or in an alternative industry. Many nursing associates have vast amounts of life and work experience, which is extremely valuable in making connections with our patients. One of the key differences between HCSWs and nursing associates is that HCSWs with lots of experience know *what* they are doing within their scope of practice, but nursing associates understand *why*. The 'Understanding the theory' boxes will help you to develop your understanding of theory. Reading theory can seem daunting if you have not engaged with it much in the past; however, these learning features aim to break down those barriers, build your confidence and make theory feel more accessible.

However, having a good understanding of theory can only get you so far. If you would like to be a gold standard practitioner, you will need to be able to apply theory to clinical practice. The case studies throughout the book will help you to do this. Based on real-life stories, case studies are written examples of what can happen in clinical practice. There may be an activity following a case study that provides you with an opportunity to write a summary of what your actions would be if you were working as a nursing associate in the case study. There are not necessarily perfect answers to activities, but there are often outline answers provided at the end of the chapters, and you can self-assess your ideas against these suggestions. A word of caution: be honest with yourself. It is paramount that you identify what you have done well and how you could improve what you have written – there is seldom such a thing as perfection in our profession. All names used in the case studies are pseudonyms and the storylines have been altered to ensure that confidentiality is maintained.

Towards the end of the book, there is a glossary of key terms, which are highlighted in **bold** the first time they are used in the book. You may wish to consider creating your own glossary of key terms and their definitions to help you remember terminology. Remember to adjust your communication methods appropriately and to avoid professional jargon when having conversations with patients.

Terminology

Throughout this book, the term 'patient' has been used. It is acknowledged that in some clinical settings, the term 'patient' may not be the most suitable. Some people interpret a patient to be unwell. However, a pregnant woman is not unwell (and therefore, not a patient), she is just pregnant. 'Service user' is another term you may hear that refers to someone using a health and/or social care service. Some people prefer to avoid being labelled as this because it makes them feel that they are dependent on the service, when in fact an objective is to promote their independence. For the purposes of this book and to provide consistency, the term 'patient' has been used to encompass all references and synonyms of this term.

A final note

This book is intended to be a foundation stone of your practice. It does not provide you with everything you need to know about person-centred care, but it points you in the right direction and is something you can come back to throughout your career. You are encouraged to challenge your own practice, strive to be the best nursing associate you can be, and demonstrate to professionals and patients how you make a positive contribution to person-centred care. Remember, you are part of a new profession, and not everyone understands what a nursing associate is yet. If someone questions you, appreciate their curiosity and tell them what it means to be a nursing associate – explain the diverse, adaptable and person-centred role you have within the MDT.

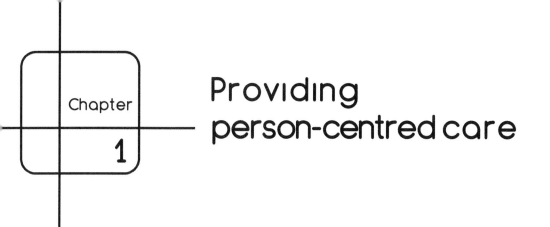

Providing person-centred care

Chapter aims

After reading this chapter, you will be able to:

- identify the predominant milestones in the NHS's history, as well as describing how they have shaped the modern NHS and the formation of the nursing associate profession;
- list the members of the multidisciplinary team (MDT) and explain the role of a nursing associate in relation to person-centred care and the wider MDT;
- define and understand the core principles of person-centred care in relation to your role as a nursing associate;
- use a variety of tools to have a sense of self-awareness, as well as the impact that your personal characteristics have on patient care.

Introduction

Nursing associates are the newest profession to join the Nursing and Midwifery Council (NMC) register. Many healthcare practitioners and members of the public may not yet have an in-depth understanding of what nursing associates are and what they can do. Imagine someone asks, 'You're a nursing associate? What's that?' This question could have a very simple answer; however, as you begin to explain that a nursing associate is someone who cares for patients, I am sure you will agree that there is more to your story.

In this chapter, we are going to discuss the heritage of the NHS and learn how this has led to the formation of the nursing associate profession. Having an awareness of your professional history will enable you to confidently discuss with colleagues, patients and the public what it means to be a nursing associate. Moreover, it will consolidate your understanding of your role in providing person-centred care.

Person-centred care is a broad subject, hence the diverse content of this book. A good starting point is to understand the core principles of person-centred care and how this improves the quality of care for patients. During this chapter, you will gain an insight into these principles and learn how to apply them in your practice. However, every practitioner is different. Diversity in the health and social care workforce is a representation of the patients we care for – no two people are the same. Your life experience and background make you a unique practitioner. Of course, we strive for standardised, high-quality person-centred care across the NHS; however, having a higher level of self-awareness will improve your understanding of how you, as an individual, have a positive impact on providing person-centred care. This is what you will uncover by the end of this chapter.

A brief history of the NHS

The NHS was originally established to provide healthcare that was free at the point of delivery (NHS, 2018a). The idea was that if people maintained good health, their reliance on acute services would be minimal. In other words, people would only need to use secondary healthcare services (such as hospitals) when they were severely unwell. The NHS was the first organisation in the world to provide such a service with zero cost at the point of delivery. Since its establishment on 5 July 1948, however, the NHS has undergone several changes and the patient population it serves is very different. Table 1.1 is a timeline of significant events that have happened in the history of the NHS.

Table 1.1   Timeline of the NHS

Decade	What happened?	Why is this important for nursing associates providing person-centred care?
1940s	• 1948: Establishment of the NHS by the then Minister of Health, Aneurin Bevan.	The original three core principles of the NHS still guide its development today: • that it meets the needs of everyone; • that it be free at the point of delivery; • that it be based on clinical need, not ability to pay.
1950s	• 1954: Sir Richard Doll and Sir Austin Bradford Hill published a paper in the *British Medical Journal (BMJ)* stating that there was a link between smoking and cancer. At this time, 80 per cent of the adult population in the UK were smokers. • 1955: Polio vaccination introduced. • 1957: The Percy Report advised the government that, where possible, people with mental healthcare needs should be cared for in the community, not in large institutions. • 1959: The Mental Health Act 1959 laid out that people with mental healthcare needs should be considered equal to those with physical healthcare needs, and care should be community-based.	The 1950s was a pivotal moment in promoting good health with the introduction of vaccinations and the recognition that smoking was linked to cancer. Mental healthcare finally got the recognition it deserved, and patients were cared for more appropriately.
1960s	• 1962: Enoch Powell's hospital plan served as a framework for the development of district general hospitals for populations of approximately 125,000 people.	The establishment of district general hospitals marked a point in time when the NHS needed to adapt to care for an increasing population.
1970s	• 1972: Computerised tomography (CT) scanners were introduced to provide 3D images of inside the human body, supporting medical diagnosis.	Technology began to play an important part in patient care.

(Continued)

Table 1.1   (Continued)

Decade	What happened?	Why is this important for nursing associates providing person-centred care?
1980s	• 1980: The Black Report recognised health inequalities. • 1985: The Whitehall II study investigated the effects of socio-economic factors on health and wellbeing, involving 10,000 civil servants.	The Black Report was formal recognition that there were health inequalities in the country. This was consolidated by the Whitehall II study, which found evidence that the socio-economic backgrounds of people affected their health. Whitehall II is still ongoing at University College London and is a well-known study of the ageing process.
1990s	• 1990: The NHS Community Care Act 1990 disbanded the centralised NHS into 57 NHS trusts, meaning that health authorities managed their own budgets to serve their local populations.	The NHS Community Care Act 1990 was another paradigm shift to serve an even larger population and attempt to manage the accompanying financial demands.
2000s	• 2000: The four-hour target for A&E was established, covering arrival to transfer, admission or discharge. • 2009: The NHS Constitution was published and the Care Quality Commission (CQC) was launched.	The use of A&E services was greater than ever before, so the four-hour target was introduced to speed up the flow of patients through emergency departments. The NHS Constitution is the most current document explaining the values of the NHS, whereas the CQC inspects the quality of health and social care services.
2010s	• 2012: The Health and Social Care Act 2012 established NHS England and Public Health England (PHE), as well as ending primary care trusts (PCTs) and introducing clinical commissioning groups (CCGs) to manage the finances of local services. • 2013: The Francis Report exposed the failings of Mid Staffordshire NHS Trust after an in-depth investigation. • 2013: The Cavendish Review found that health and social care support workers need better education and support.	The two reports published in the 2010s were extensive and shook the modern NHS. The system failed patients, and the recommendations made were to prevent such a catastrophe from happening again. Notably, funding for education for healthcare support workers was dramatically increased. The financial system was reorganised again. The executive management was divided into NHS England for patient services and PHE to promote health and well being.

Source: BHF (2018)

Now that you have read about some significant events that have happened in the history of the NHS, complete Activity 1.1, which will help you to explain and understand how the history of the NHS has shaped the nursing associate profession in the present day.

Activity 1.1   Critical thinking

Think about how the significant events in each decade of the NHS timeline in Table 1.1 affected patient care. Make a list of each decade and identify the connections between events in each decade and the NMC *Standards of Proficiency for Nursing Associates*.

An outline answer is provided at the end of the chapter.

The modern NHS

In the present day, the NHS is one of the largest employers in the world, not to mention the largest and oldest healthcare service. The management system is complex, which reflects the scale of the NHS at large. Table 1.2 outlines different micro-organisations that contribute to maintaining the standards of the NHS, outlined in the NHS Constitution (NHS England, 2015b).

Table 1.2   Structure of the NHS management system

Department of Health and Social Care (DHSC)	The DHSC advises the government on national health and social care policy and provides direction for the NHS. It also decides on how the total NHS budget is divided up. The majority of the money is sent to NHS England.
NHS England	NHS England is the management head of the NHS (not the government). It commissions NHS services and sets strategies at a national level. Most money is transferred to CCGs.
Clinical commissioning groups (CCGs)	There are over 200 CCGs in England. They identify health and social care needs in their local areas, then fund the services to meet those needs. These services include NHS trusts, the private sector, GP surgeries, mental health services, charities and community services.
NHS Improvement (NHSI)	NHSI oversees the operational management of NHS trusts, predominantly the finances, and provides advice on how to improve services from a national perspective.
Care Quality Commission (CQC)	The CQC conducts inspections of NHS trusts and other health and social care agencies. It assesses how each organisation is performing in relation to a set of standards. Each organisation is graded using a traffic light colour system, and the results are openly published.
National Institute for Health and Care Excellence (NICE)	NICE completes research studies into a wide variety of topics and produces guidance for NHS trusts and clinicians. Each organisation bases their policies on NICE guidance, but they may adapt their policies to meet the needs of the local populations they serve.
Health Education England (HEE)	HEE leads all education and training for the NHS health and social care workforce. It commissions different programmes on national and regional scales and reports directly to the DHSC. It also led the national pilot and implementation of the nursing associate profession.
Nursing and Midwifery Council (NMC)	The NMC is the governing body of all UK nurses, midwives and nursing associates. It is responsible for protecting the public and maintaining the high standards of the nursing and midwifery professions.
Royal College of Nursing (RCN)	The RCN is a large trade union of the nursing professions and is a membership organisation. It is the representative body of the nursing and midwifery workforce, and aims to support, protect and celebrate these professions. Nursing associate are welcome to join the RCN and receive the same benefits as the other nursing professions.

Source: DHSC (2018)

As a nursing associate, it is important for you to have an understanding of the micro-organisations that manage the NHS because the decisions they make directly affect your clinical practice. Complete Activity 1.2 to consolidate your understanding.

Activity 1.2   Reflection

Rearrange the list in Table 1.2 into a thought cloud, starting with the NHS in the middle. Link all the different micro-organisations together to illustrate how the NHS management system is structured.

As this activity is based on your own reflection, there is no outline answer provided at the end of the chapter.

After completing Activity 1.2, you will have a clearer picture of how the NHS is managed. Your thought cloud may look complex, but this is a true representation of the systems in place that ensure the NHS meets the standards described in the NHS Constitution (DHSC, 2015). At this point, you have learned about the NHS's past and present, but what about the future?

What is next?

Across England, there are trials of new systems of health and social care services, called vanguard sites. Vanguard sites aim to encourage organisations to work more closely together, including the collaboration of physical and mental healthcare needs, in sustainability and transformation partnerships (STPs). STPs are groups of organisations that work together to achieve the objective of vanguard sites; there are 44 in England. STPs aim to transition into integrated care systems (ICSs). ICSs work together with a joined budget to coordinate care and improve services for people who live in a particular community. In short, ICSs aim to manage the limited resources of the NHS more efficiently and provide continuity of care across their organisations' services. This involves working with other bodies, such as local authorities, social care services and public health organisations, in order to drive up standards of service.

What does all of this change mean for patients? Some services in the NHS are moving closer to patients to provide the care they need where most people would choose to be – at home. There is a substantial increase in support to improve and maintain good health, thus reducing the intense pressure on hospital services (King's Fund, 2017). There are, however, some points for consideration. Regional health specialist services will become more common, which means that patients may need to travel further for specialised care. Moreover, the NHS will need to continue to change over the next few decades. Although more change may seem arduous, change is very much needed in the NHS because our patients continue to change. As a nation, we are living longer, with more complex care needs, so NHS services need to be able to meet new patient needs. Make sure you keep up to date with how the NHS is managed and the services that it provides throughout your career, as this will have an impact on your future as a nursing associate. See Chapter 8 for advice on how to keep your practice up to date and current.

The multidisciplinary team

The NHS is clearly complex, but where do nursing associates fit in this system? A **multidisciplinary team** (MDT) is a group of health and social care professionals who work together to provide care for patients. You are part of this team and have a unique, important role. Before going into which professionals make up an MDT, we need to discuss what a professional is.

Being a professional is more than doing a good job. As a nursing associate, you are a health and social care professional, but what does this actually mean? There are many attributes of a health and social care professional that are important for you to understand. Professionals' behaviour is of a consistently high standard, even when not at work. Being a professional is also about being in a professional community: we have common values and morals, we always strive to do our very best in everything we do, and we always continue to learn and adapt our practice. All of this is done in the best interests of the patients we care for. Table 1.3 lists important key documents that guide you in being a professional, with a short explanation of how they do this.

Table 1.3   Key documents

The Code (NMC, 2018b)	The standards of clinical practice and behaviour that are expected of all nurses, midwives and nursing associates.
Leading Change, Adding Value (NHS England, 2016)	A framework of ten commitments that guide the NHS workforce to provide the best quality person-centred care.
The NHS Constitution (DHSC, 2015)	This document explains the values of the NHS, including what patients and employees can expect from the service.

It can sometimes be hard to understand how overarching policy documents such as these relate directly to your practice as a nursing associate. To help you understand this, read through the following box, which breaks down each document and explains how it is relevant to your daily practice.

Understanding the theory: key documents

The Code (NMC, 2018b)

This document is fundamental to your practice, and you are encouraged to know it in depth. There are four sections that guide your clinical practice: 'Prioritise people', 'Practise effectively', 'Preserve safety', and 'Promote professionalism and trust'. Another important document closely linked to *The Code* is the *Standards of Proficiency for Nursing Associates* (NMC, 2018a). Take the time to read this too because it outlines your scope of practice.

Leading Change, Adding Value (NHS England, 2016)

The 'Leading change' section is grouped into three topics: 'Health and wellbeing', 'Care and quality', and 'Funding and efficiency'. As a nursing associate, you can positively contribute to all of these. First, it is part of your scope of practice to promote health and wellbeing for patients in your care. Second, you use evidence-based practice to provide person-centred care (see later in this chapter). Lastly, by using resources effectively and efficiently, you will reduce

(Continued)

(Continued)

the expenditure of the area you work in, and by extension the NHS. By doing these three things, you will reduce **unwarranted variation**, which minimises the things we do not want to happen (people becoming more ill and then receiving poor standards of care, which costs a lot of money). The 'Adding value' section explains how you can achieve better outcomes, better experiences and a better use of resources for patients by consistently demonstrating the 6Cs: care, compassion, competence, communication, courage and commitment.

The NHS Constitution (DHSC, 2015)

The foremost message is that the NHS belongs to the British public. Both patients and practitioners have a vested interest, and this document explains this. The guiding principles of the NHS are outlined, as well as the NHS's values. The rights of patients and the pledges the NHS has made are also defined in the NHS Constitution. Without NHS staff, there would be no service, so staff rights and responsibilities are also included.

A good way to assess your own practice and check that you are maintaining the standards of the health and social care profession is to ask yourself throughout your day, 'If this was being filmed, would I edit the film before showing it to my manager?' If your answer is 'no', you can be confident that you are acting with professional **integrity**.

Now that you have an understanding of what it means to be a professional, let us look at an MDT in more detail. Any MDT will meet to plan the necessary care for a patient they are all caring for. If possible, it is recommended that the patient attends this meeting too because, after all, they are why the MDT is meeting. Table 1.4 lists the professionals who may be involved in an MDT. This will depend on the patient's needs and the clinical environment they are in (i.e. at home, a close-to-home service or in hospital). Table 1.4 is not an extensive list, nor does it mean that every professional mentioned needs to be involved in an MDT – it all depends on the situation. It may seem like a lot of people; however, each profession meets different patients' needs. Only the professionals who have an input in the patient's care are present at the MDT. Each patient (and their needs) is different, so each MDT will have different professionals present.

Table 1.4   Professionals in the MDT

Doctor	The medical lead of the MDT who has extensive knowledge on diagnosis and the treatment needed.
Nurse	The holistic care lead and advocate for the patient.
Occupational therapist	Assesses and works with patients to achieve their potential in both physical and mental health, in a safe environment.
Physiotherapist	Supports patients to maintain and improve their physical health needs.
Healthcare support worker (HCSW)	Provides fundamental care to patients and supports the nursing, physiotherapist and occupational therapist professions.
Dietician	Qualified to assess, diagnose and manage issues with diet and nutrition.
Nutritionist	An expert who provides advice on nutritional benefits to health.
Speech and language therapist	Provides treatment and support to adults and children with communication, eating, drinking and swallowing issues.
Nursing associate	A generalist practitioner that can work in all fields of nursing (adult, paediatric, mental health and learning disability) across the lifespan.

Source: NHS England (2015a)

Attending an MDT meeting for the first time can make some people feel anxious because there might be a lot of people in the room. However, it is important to remember that everyone in the MDT is there to support each other, as well as supporting the patient in achieving their goals. Once you have been to a few MDT meetings, you will gain more confidence, and eventually you may contribute to the discussions. Whether you have been to one or many, attending an MDT meeting is a very useful learning opportunity because you gain an insight into the roles of other professions, as well as how they have a positive impact through providing person-centred care.

Once you have attended an MDT meeting, complete Activity 1.3 to consolidate what you have learned. Do not limit yourself to completing this activity once, though. Each MDT meeting you attend will be different, so you can learn something new from each meeting you attend.

Activity 1.3   Reflection

After attending an MDT meeting, think about your answers to the following questions:

1. What was the role of each professional who attended the meeting?
2. If the patient attended, how did this affect the meeting? If the patient did not attend, how do you think the meeting might have gone differently if the patient was present?
3. What were the strengths and achievements of the meeting?
4. How could the meeting have been improved?

As this activity is based on your own reflection, there is no outline answer provided at the end of the chapter.

As previously discussed, the main aim of an MDT is to meet patients' needs. At this point in the chapter, you will be able to recognise that each patient is different and their needs unique, even if a group of patients have the same diagnosis. In other words, the MDT cannot care for patients using generic principles because this would not meet individual patients' needs. A person-centred approach to care, however, ensures that each patient is cared for as an individual and their needs are met.

What is person-centred care?

Every registered practitioner and support worker that has direct or indirect patient contact should **critically analyse** the positive and negative impacts of their decisions to ensure that all NHS services operate with a person-centred approach. It is also important to emphasise the phrase 'each patient'. While we can group patients together by many different characteristics, such as age, sex or the condition they are living with, it is important to remember that each person is unique, even identical twins. These differences occur due to our genetics, the environments in which we live and our life experiences. The influencing factors that cause these differences can be explained by the **social determinants of health**, which are summarised in the following box.

Understanding the theory: social determinants of health

Originally published in the seminal article by Dahlgren and Whitehead (1991), PHE (2017) explains that the social determinants of health are:

- genetic and personal factors;
- lifestyle choices;
- interpersonal relationships with family, friends and the community;
- living and employment conditions:
  - food production;
  - education;
  - work environment;
  - unemployment;
  - water and sanitation management;
  - health and social care services;
  - housing;
- general socio-economic, cultural and environmental conditions.

Quite simply, these influencing factors are what determines the health and wellbeing of a patient, as well as what makes them unique. Two patients sitting next to each other will have completely different backgrounds in relation to their social determinants of health, so it is impossible to care for them in exactly the same way, even if they may have the same health concern. It is therefore important to understand the different social determinants of health, as understanding these for each of your patients will enable you to deliver effective person-centred care.

To explore the ideas outlined in the previous box, it may be of benefit to examine a specific example of a health condition. The following case study is based on a patient living with the common long-term condition asthma.

Case study: George

George is a 27-year-old man who has had asthma since early childhood. When he has an asthma attack, he finds it difficult to breathe and has an audible wheeze. What causes George's asthma attacks are known as asthmatic triggers, some examples of which are animal fur, cold air, dust, exercise, pollen and sress. Not all of these asthmatic triggers need to be present to cause an asthma attack, and furthermore each person living with asthma has a different response to asthmatic triggers. To control his asthma attacks, George self-administers his salbutamol inhaler, following the instructions written on the prescription.

It is impossible to write down an algorithm that determines which asthmatic triggers will cause an asthma attack because everyone is sensitive to asthmatic triggers at different severity levels. Some people may be sensitive to one specific asthmatic trigger, such as long-haired tabby cats, while others may not. In other words, health and social care practitioners must care for each patient differently. It is more accurate to say that each health and social care practitioner must care for each patient *specifically*. This proves the point that nursing associates must also practise with a person-centred care approach in order to meet patients' specific needs. If this does not happen, the patient will not receive the correct care, and they may become more unwell or begin to deteriorate.

The above case study leads on to another important point: knowing what to do to care for patients. Historically, health and social care was based on traditional practice. Traditional practice meant passing down anecdotal methods of how to care for patients, such as how to treat a wound. The theory behind this was that traditional practice passed the test of time – it has been done a certain way for many years, and so it does not need to change. This is dangerous and puts patients at risk. There should be a red flag waving inside your head if you hear someone say, 'That's the way we've always done it here', or words to that effect. We will come on to how to manage that situation soon, but first we need to look at what you should base your practice on. You will read the term '**evidence-based practice**' a lot throughout health and social care literature. The reason that traditional practice puts patients at risk is that the methods have not been tested to check if they produce the best outcome for the patient. The worst-case scenario is that traditional practice intervention may cause the patient greater harm. An example of this is the historic method of applying butter to treat burns. This was considered normal practice at one time. However, if we think about it, butter is a fat that we can melt to cook things. Considering that a burn is hot, when butter was applied, it melted and continued to burn the patient, making the wound worse than it was before. This sounds obvious from the perspective of the present day but is an example of traditional practice that was common for many years. Evidence-based practice, however, is founded on testing an intervention to see if it works before using it to care for patients.

Evidence-based practice is produced from **research** studies. A research study is a project that systematically investigates if a clinical or therapeutic intervention has the best outcome for the patient. A **systematic** investigation means that there is a strict method in the project, which is clearly explained in the write-up and could be repeated by following those instructions. A research study also needs to be valid and trustworthy. To achieve this, researchers outline how they have attempted to control the influencing factors that could alter the results of the study, as well as declaring the limitations of the study. A research study that investigates the benefit of a new dressing to treat burns which involved one adult male participant is not representative of the patient population, and would hence be considered to have limited transferability to clinical practice. *The Code* states that nursing associates are required to be able to read and comprehend research papers, as well as local trust policies, to base their practice on (NMC, 2018b). By doing this, you will be providing evidence-based care, and thus reducing the risk of harm to the patient. Risk cannot be totally removed because each patient is different, but it can be reduced and mitigated by using evidence-based practice. The risk in traditional practice is uncontrolled; therefore, evidence-based practice is always what you should base your clinical and therapeutic practice on.

So, what should you do if you hear that remark mentioned earlier, 'That's the way we've always done it here'? You are likely to hear words to that effect if you ask why you should use a certain intervention to care for a patient. This is a perfectly reasonable question for you to ask, but remember you may be working in a highly stressful, pressured environment or situation. Choose carefully when and where you ask questions; unless a patient's safety is at risk, asking a question in a private room without an audience is much more professional and considerate. To learn about the rationale (and evidence) behind an intervention, you could word your question as follows: 'I've not seen this intervention before. I'm interested to know the evidence base behind it. Please could we go through it together?' You can adapt this wording to suit the situation you are in; however, by asking the question in this way, you are demonstrating that you have professional curiosity, and the person you are speaking with is less likely to misinterpret you and feel you are being accusatory. In short, you are promoting teamwork and a learning culture in the area you are in. This has massive benefits for staff because people then feel they can ask questions and develop their practice. Moreover, patients benefit because the staff are working together to provide evidence-based care. Think back to earlier in this chapter when it was outlined that person-centred care means we critically analyse the positive and negative impacts on each patient we care for. By adopting this approach, you are thinking about the impact on the patients you are caring for, and therefore demonstrating person-centred care.

Self-awareness

Person-centred care is not solely about knowing your patient and what makes them an individual; you also need to know yourself. More specifically, you need to know and understand how you have an impact on the patient. The impact you make may be very positive; however, you must be cautious of making a negative impact on the patient. As you have been reading, each patient is unique because of their social determinants of health. Social determinants of health help us to understand each patient's individuality in relation to their health; however, they can also help us to understand patients' personalities. This also applies to you. Nursing associates can be patients, of course, but the more pressing point here is that your background defines you as a person, and by extension informs the choices you make and the personality you have. Your approach to a task may be completely different to that of one of your colleagues who completed the apprenticeship with you, despite the fact that you both studied at the same institution. Activity 1.4 explores this in a little more detail.

Activity 1.4   Reflection

Consider how you approach writing an academic essay. Do you leave it all to the last minute, needing the pressure of an impending deadline? Or do you prefer to follow the recommended route of creating a structured study plan, completing the essay comfortably before the deadline, because you find this is a better way to manage your stress levels? Compare your thoughts with friends and colleagues. You may recognise that you are all completing the same task but have very different methods.

As this activity is based on your own reflection, there is no outline answer provided at the end of the chapter.

How do your reflections in Activity 1.4 relate to person-centred care? Consider the responses you received from your friends and colleagues, and how differently they interpreted the standardised process of writing an academic essay. Imagine the diversity of interpretations in the varied and high-pressured environment of clinical practice. The way that you and your colleagues approach any task will inevitably be different. It is positive to have professional individuality because a diverse workforce is a reflection of the patients we care for; however, it is important to mitigate against possible negative effects on a patient. This should help you to understand why having increased self-awareness of your own strengths, weaknesses and preferences will help you and your colleagues to provide the best quality person-centred care.

Diversity in the NHS workforce is clearly beneficial; however, let us refocus on how you can have an even greater positive impact on person-centred care. Working as a nursing associate is a privilege because you are in a position to care for people when they are at their most vulnerable, and they trust you to do so. We must recognise, however, that working as a nursing associate can be stressful and emotive due to the high pressure of caring for people when they are vulnerable. This leads on to another important point: you need to be continually conscious of your attitudes and behaviours because they affect other people. In other words, allowing yourself to choose a negative outlook will cause your colleagues and patients to do the same. Alternatively, actively ensuring that you have a positive attitude and behaviour will encourage others to adopt the same approach. This can be a very powerful force for good, especially if you meet a patient or colleague having a bad day. (It is worth remembering that it is likely your patients will almost always be having a worse day than you.) Read through the following box to help you understand how your attitudes and behaviours affect other people.

Understanding the theory: Betari's box

Betari's box is a tool you can use to illustrate how your own thoughts and actions have an effect on other people (Mind Tools, 2019a). This could be your colleagues, your patients, or even your friends and family after you arrive home from work. First, you need to identify your attitudes, which are determined by your feelings and/or prejudices. Next, you need to identify how your attitudes affect your behaviour. A note of caution: you must be honest with yourself about your behaviour. For example, you may naturally have strong facial expressions, so your thoughts and feelings are obvious to those around you. Ask a genuine friend or colleague if you are not sure. Your attitudes and behaviours then lead on to affect another person's attitude. Lastly, the way you have affected someone's attitude affects their behaviour. If you apply the process in Betari's box to a clinical practice setting, you will be able to recognise if your attitudes and behaviours have a positive or negative effect on other people. In other words, your attitudes and behaviours may alter a patient's attitudes and behaviours, which could lead to them making the wrong decision or feeling worse. A positive example would be actively listening to a patient who is depressed and demonstrating empathy, which may elevate their mood, thus supporting them in managing their depression.

Regularly completing the process outlined in Betari's box will help you to be mindful of your attitudes and behaviours throughout your career, as well as encouraging you to channel positivity into your clinical practice. Having consistently positive attitudes and behaviours will encourage others to have the same approach, including both your colleagues and patients. Positivity leads to an increase in efficiency and effectiveness, so the quality of patient care will increase. By choosing to practise in this way, you are choosing to promote person-centred care.

Chapter summary

This chapter has provided you with an insight into the history of the NHS, and you will have recognised how significant events in the history of the NHS have informed the nursing associate profession in the present day. Remember to keep yourself up to date with changes in the NHS and the management systems in place; change is inevitable because our patients are changing, and we need to ensure that we are providing person-centred care at all times to meet their needs. The importance of nursing associate practice, as well as how it compares to other members of the MDT, has also been discussed. Each profession within the MDT will be focused on meeting a specific need of a patient, but what makes nursing associates unique is their generalist approach to person-centred care across the lifespan and in the context of all four fields of nursing. After reading this chapter, you will now have a more consolidated understanding of the core principles of person-centred care in relation to your clinical practice as a nursing associate. Lastly, you now have more in-depth understanding and self-awareness about how you can positively contribute to ensuring person-centred care.

Activities: Brief outline answers

Activity 1.1 Critical thinking (page 11)

The events that took place during the history of the NHS in each decade have direct links with the platforms of the NMC *Standards of Proficiency for Nursing Associates*. There may be more than one link to a platform for each decade; but here are some suggestions that you can use to self-assess your list:

- 1940s: Platform 1: Being an accountable professional
- 1950s: Platform 2: Promoting health and preventing ill health
- 1960s: Platform 6: Contributing to integrated care
- 1970s: Platform 3: Provide and monitor care
- 1980s: Platform 5: Improving safety and quality of care
- 1990s: Platform 4: Working in teams
- 2000s: Platform 1: Being an accountable professional
- 2010s: Platform 5: Improving safety and quality of care

Annotated further reading

de Bono, E. (2016) *Six Thinking Hats*. London: Penguin.

To learn more about your strengths and areas of development in relation to how you approach tasks and think, read this seminal book by Edward de Bono. You may also be able to find alternative activities online that will help you to identify which coloured hats you wear in certain situations.

NHS England (2015) *MDT Development*. Available at: www.england.nhs.uk/wp-content/uploads/2015/01/mdt-dev-guid-flat-fin.pdf

For more information about MDTs and the meetings they have, read this publication by NHS England.

Price, B. (2019) *Delivering Person-Centred Care in Nursing.* London: SAGE.

This book is an excellent introduction to person-centred care that has comprehensive content and a clear structure. Although it is intended for nursing students, much of the material is also relevant to nursing associate practice.

Willis, P. (2015) *Shape of Caring Review (Raising the Bar).* Available at: www.hee.nhs.uk/our-work/shape-caring-review

This is the publication of an extensive review into the education and professional development of nursing and healthcare support workers following the Mid Staffordshire NHS Trust scandal.

Useful websites

16Personalities Free Personality Test: www.16personalities.com/free-personality-test

For an in-depth insight into your personality and characteristics, this website provides a free test based on the work of Myers and Briggs, which will help you to identify your strengths and areas for improvement.

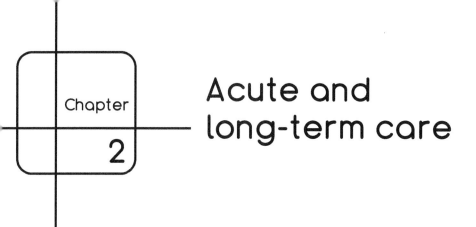

Acute and long-term care

Chapter 2

Chapter aims

After reading this chapter, you will be able to:

- use a systematic assessment method to recognise the different needs of patients with acute and long-term conditions;
- identify patients' needs across their lifespan;
- understand person-centred care in relation to the four fields of nursing;
- develop the varied interpersonal skills needed to provide person-centred care for patients with acute and long-term conditions alongside registered nurses.

Introduction

As a nursing associate, you have a broad scope of practice that can be implemented to meet the needs of patients in any setting. You need to be able to care for people across their lifespan and in the context of all four fields of nursing: adult, paediatric, mental health and learning disability. Nursing associates are generalist practitioners, which makes them unique in comparison to the four fields of nursing and the MDT. This chapter will provide you with the tools that you need to provide person-centred care in a wide variety of clinical environments for a very diverse patient population. You will be able to achieve the aims of this chapter by engaging with the learning features found throughout, including activities, case studies and 'Understanding the theory' boxes. You will be able to find outline answers at the end of the chapter, as well as an annotated list of further reading and a list of useful websites. Patient diversity was discussed in Chapter 1, and one key learning point was that nursing associates need to be able to provide person-centred care because each patient is different. There are too many conditions that patients could have to list, but all of them can be identified as either an **acute condition** or a **long-term condition** ('long-term' is also known as 'chronic').

What does acute mean, however? How long does a condition need to last before it is identified as a long-term condition? In short, an acute condition is a sudden deterioration in the patient's health, physically or psychologically, that is usually reversible if the appropriate treatment is provided. In comparison, a long-term condition is a physical or psychological condition that has no cure. A long-term condition may improve over time, remain stable or become progressively worse. If a long-term condition does suddenly deteriorate, it is known as an exacerbation. In other words, an exacerbation of a long-term condition then becomes an acute condition. Diabetes is a relevant example.

Diabetes is a long-term condition that affects a patient's ability to produce the hormone insulin from the pancreas to control glucose levels in their blood. Type 2 diabetes is the most common type of diabetes, usually caused as a result of poor lifestyle choices (particularly unbalanced diet, sedentary lifestyle and smoking) over a long period of time. Type 1 diabetes is a **hereditary** condition, usually diagnosed in childhood. For Type 1 diabetes, patients need insulin injections, or they can wear an insulin-releasing patch that ensures their glucose levels are controlled. Patients with Type 2 diabetes may be able to manage their diabetes with a balanced diet and regular exercise. Some patients with Type 2 diabetes, however, may be prescribed a medicine called metformin or they may also need insulin (NICE, 2019). As you can see, diabetes is a long-term condition with multiple subcategories that require different interventions of care. If a patient's diabetes becomes unstable, however, they may have a hypoglycaemic attack. This is when the capillary blood glucose (CBG) level drops below 4.0 mmol/L. This is very serious because the patient's **metabolism** will not function correctly. If a hypoglycaemic attack is not treated with a source of simple glucose (e.g. a sugary drink) followed by complex carbohydrates that break down into sugar slowly (e.g. toast), the patient could become unconscious, which will lead to a diabetes-induced coma. A hypoglycaemic attack is known as an acute condition. The following case study illustrates a real-life example of how a patient can have both acute and long-term conditions.

Case study: Alice

Alice is a 58-year-old business manager in a large technology company. She has worked for the company for nearly 20 years and is a senior member of staff with many responsibilities. Three years ago, she was diagnosed with a cardiac condition called angina. Her cardiologist explained that angina is the narrowing of the coronary arteries that supply oxygenated blood to the heart muscle (**myocardium**). The narrowing of the arteries is caused by atheroma, the gradual build-up of fatty deposits in the artery walls. She explains to her cardiologist that she often eats takeaway food for both lunch and dinner because it is convenient and allows her more time to work, rather than cooking. Her cardiologist explains that the chest pain she has been experiencing is caused by insufficient blood flow to her heart when her blood pressure is raised due to exercise or stress. Alice is concerned by her diagnosis, but the cardiologist reassures her that if she makes positive lifestyle choices with her diet and starts to do regular exercise, she will be able to control her angina.

Alice decides to change her diet. She starts to prepare nutritious meals for lunch and cook home-made food for dinner, and on Fridays she goes out to a restaurant with her partner as an end of week treat. Her workload, however, starts to become unmanageable. She does her best to meet the company directors' expectations but starts to have episodes of severe chest pain again. On one occasion, the pain is so intense that her colleague calls an ambulance and Alice is brought to her local A&E. Her vital signs are measured by the nursing associate and she is reviewed by the medical registrar. The medical registrar diagnoses Alice with an angina attack and prescribes a medication called glyceryl trinitrate (GTN) that stops the chest pain.

Alice is referred back to her cardiologist for a review. The cardiologist explains that an angina attack is an acute condition that can be managed by administering GTN. The correct method is to spray the medication twice under the tongue so that it is quickly absorbed into the bloodstream. Alice learns that the GNT relaxes the smooth muscle cells in her coronary arteries, causing them to dilate and allow oxygenated blood to flow to the myocardium more easily, thus stopping the pain. The cardiologist explains that an angina attack is an exacerbation of her long-term condition, angina. The cardiologist recommends that Alice books an appointment with her workplace's occupational health department for support on how to reduce her workload so she is not constantly stressed. This will reduce the risk of her having an angina attack, providing she continues with the positive lifestyle changes she has already made.

Alice's case study demonstrates that a patient can have both acute and long-term conditions. Acute and long-term conditions change over time as a result of many influencing factors. In Chapter 8, you will read about how you can provide person-centred health promotion to help patients manage their long-term conditions, but for now complete Activity 2.1 to consolidate your understanding of acute and long-term conditions.

Activity 2.1   Reflection

The patients you care for often have a number of **co-morbidities**, which can include both acute and long-term conditions (e.g. Alice in the previous case study had angina and chronic stress). The next time you are in clinical practice caring for a patient, identify (in your head) which of their conditions are acute and which are long-term. Think about the differences in the care they may need for each of these conditions. Have a reflective discussion afterwards with your supervisor or the registered nurse you are working with to check your thoughts.

As this activity is based on your own reflection, there is no outline answer provided at the end of the chapter.

Whether a patient you are caring for has an acute or long-term condition, you will need to complete an assessment in order to establish what their needs are. This assessment must be thorough, and it goes without saying that you cannot overlook or miss anything which is potentially significant. To reduce the risk of this happening, you need to use a systematic patient assessment tool; this is a step-by-step guide when assessing patients that will help you to identify what their needs are. Remember that as a nursing associate, you should always provide person-centred care, which includes all aspects of patients' needs. In other words, you should provide holistic person-centred care. The next section looks at some of the reliable assessment tools that you can use in your clinical practice.

Systematic patient assessments

There are many different assessment tools that you can use in your clinical practice. Some are used in specific situations, whereas others are generic. The nursing process is a tool that can be applied to any patient, in any clinical environment, at any stage of their lifespan. Considering that you will be working with patients across their lifespan and in any of the four fields of nursing, the nursing process is very useful for you because it is has high **generalisation** value. In other words, the nursing process can be used as your guide, which can be of great support to you if you are working in a new clinical area and are unsure what you are expected to be doing. To learn more about the nursing process, read the following box.

Understanding the theory: the nursing process

According to Howatson-Jones et al. (2015), the nursing process has five stages. You can use the nursing process to guide you through the caring process of any patient. The nursing process does not tell you specifically what to do, but it does provide high-level guidance to your practice. The steps below have been adapted for nursing associates, based on Howatson-Jones et al.'s (2015) nursing process. These can be reassuring if you are working in a new area that is unfamiliar to you.

1. Assessment

In the assessment stage, you can use a patient assessment tool to help you establish what the patient's needs are. This is the stage when you gather all the information about the patient's condition and situation. Your main role here is to identify any red flags (signs of deterioration) and what care needs the patient has, as well as being ready to communicate this succinctly to a registered nurse.

2. Patient goals

Nursing associates do not provide a diagnosis, but you can identify what the patient's primary concerns are. Another way to describe the nursing diagnosis stage of the nursing process is that you are identifying the patient's goals in relation to their health and wellbeing. They may have an immediate need, such as pain relief, or a more long-term goal, such as being able to walk independently after having a **stroke**. Always remember to escalate any concerns outside of your scope of practice to the appropriately qualified practitioner – check the *Standards of Proficiency for Nursing Associates* if you are unsure (NMC, 2018a). It is highly likely that there will be more than one goal, hence why you need to complete a thorough holistic assessment. To find out more, read the section on SMART goals later in the chapter.

3. Planning

After your assessment and establishing the patient's goals, you need to plan what you are going to do to meet the patient's needs. This may be something you, as a nursing associate, will do, or you will make a referral to another member of the MDT. If there is more than one goal, you need to put them into priority order. Later in this chapter, you will read about the A-G assessment tool, which can help you with prioritising. Remember to include in your plan a time frame for implementation and evaluation, which will be recorded in the patient's care plan. You will read about care plans later in this chapter too.

4. Implementation

This is the stage where you and other members of the MDT will put the plan into action. By doing so, you will be supporting the patient to achieve the goals that you identified in the second stage. Remember to adhere to the principles of person-centred care, as discussed in Chapter 1.

5. Evaluation

After all of the implementation steps have been completed, the final stage of the nursing process is to evaluate if the patient's goals have been achieved. If they have, great – the patient is likely to be transferred to another service or discharged. There will be times, however, when the patient's goals have not been achieved for some reason. The patient (and you) may feel frustrated by this, but remember that there are some circumstances which are out of our control. The important thing to remember at this stage is that the nursing process is cyclic, meaning you can restart at any point, at any time. It may be that the implemented care did not work for this patient on this occasion, and so a new assessment, nursing diagnosis and plan need to take place.

    The nursing process only has five stages, which has great benefits because you do not need to spend a long time remembering a complicated formula. Although the nursing process is simple and easy to remember, applying it in clinical practice will provide you with

(Continued)

(Continued)

guidance to provide person-centred care for a patient. Furthermore, the nursing process is flexible, allowing you to stop and restart at any stage. The next time you go into clinical practice, try to identify what happens for a patient at each stage of the nursing process and compare this with another patient's care. You will be able to see that the nursing process is a tool that can be applied to all clinical environments for any patient.

Whenever you care for a patient, you will subconsciously complete the first stage of the nursing process (i.e. assessment). Whether you are revisiting a patient or meeting them for the first time, you will often gain a first impression of their health and wellbeing. Have you ever looked at someone and suddenly thought, 'They do not look very well at all'? This is your clinical intuition, or first impression. It is likely that you are already able to identify your clinical intuition because there are some easily identifiable signs and symptoms to look out for when gaining a first impression of how well or unwell a patient is. Complete Activity 2.2 to help you recognise the potential stages of the thought process that you are using in your clinical intuition.

Activity 2.2   Reflection

When first meeting a patient, even if you have met them before, using your clinical intuition can help you to identify if the patient is acutely unwell or in pain, or has a different immediate care need. This activity lists four topics of different signs and symptoms that you can observe when initially meeting a patient. You may already subconsciously assess these, but reflecting on them can help you to consolidate your practice. To help you remember them, the observations have been listed as 'A to D'. You could complete this A-D assessment before moving on to the more familiar A-G assessment, which is discussed later in this chapter. The only equipment that you need for an A-D assessment is your basic observation and communication skills.

1. Appearance

Imagine that you are approaching a patient, either in a hospital or in their own home. At this stage, take note of how they appear. Make sure that you assess their appearance objectively, not subjectively. Describing a patient's appearance as 'scruffy' could have many different interpretations, or even be hurtful, whereas describing their appearance as 'partially dressed and unshaven' is **objective**. You may notice that the patient's colour is different: cyanosis (blue), flushed (red), jaundiced (yellow) or mottled (patchy colours). Be careful not to start describing their behaviour until the next stage.

2. Behaviour

As you get closer to the patient, observe their behaviour. An important question to ask yourself is, 'Is this behaviour expected and appropriate for this patient?' If the patient is acting out of character, this could be a sign that something is wrong. If you have never met the patient before, assessing their behaviour is more challenging, but you can use your intuition and common sense. For example, it is typically unusual for an elderly patient to swear at you before you have introduced yourself (although there may be exceptions, of course!). Unexpected behaviour could be a sign of an underlying acute or chronic condition, such as **delirium**. If you are still unsure, move on to the next stage to establish more information.

3. Communication

You are now likely to be next to the patient, so you need to introduce yourself. The best way to do this is by continuing the legacy of Dr Kate Granger, a consultant geriatrician who had cancer. During her treatment, she noticed that she did not know many of the healthcare staff's names, so she started a campaign called **#hellomynameis** (Granger, 2013). Dr Granger advocated that all health and social care staff should introduce themselves using 'Hello, my name is ...' so that every patient knew who was looking after them. Her legacy has spread around the world and has unquestionably improved standards of care. At this stage of your initial assessment, you can also shake the patient's hand (providing you maintain infection control precautions). By doing this, you will be able to assess the patient's warmth, strength and coordination, as well as helping to build a rapport between you and the patient.

4. Demeanour

The final stage of your initial assessment is an assessment of the patient's demeanour. You have now spent around 30 seconds gathering important information, so you will be able to identify any first impression concerns. The patient may have told you, 'I am in a lot of pain', which is evidently a high priority; however, some patients may not want to be a nuisance, and will avoid saying they are in pain, but their actions may tell you otherwise. Lastly, this is a perfect opportunity for you to ask the patient what their main concern is and what they would like you to do. Asking this question demonstrates that you are putting their concerns at the centre of your care, and hence you are demonstrating person-centred care.

The next time you are in clinical practice, see if you can identify if you are observing these items, or whether you have observed something else with a patient you are caring for. Discuss your reflection with your supervisor or line manager the next time you meet with them. Remember that your initial assessment using your clinical intuition, such as the observations listed in this activity, will inform the next part of the nursing process. If you are concerned by something or recognise that a patient is acutely unwell, call for help from your supervisor or another nearby registered practitioner to help you.

As this activity is based on your own reflection, there is no outline answer provided at the end of the chapter.

Completing an initial assessment, such as the A-D assessment in Activity 2.2, in clinical practice will inform the nursing process and your next assessment. Linking back to the nursing process, you need to choose an appropriate assessment tool in order for you to identify the patient's goals. There are many assessment tools that you can use, but your trust may advocate a particular one. A reliable and transferable tool is the A-G assessment. It is important to note that each NHS trust may have different policies and clinical guidance. For example, London NHS trusts usually use an A-G assessment tool (but there may be expeditions), whereas NHS trusts outside of London and pre-hospital care providers usually use an A-E assessment tool. Furthermore, each letter of the acronym may have slightly different meanings, so you will need to check this. This is not a case of right or wrong, but making sure that your practice adheres to the policy of the trust you are working in. In this book, the A-G assessment tool is referred to, but remember to check which version to use when you are next in clinical practice. Read the following box to find out more.

Understanding the theory: A-G assessment tool and National Early Warning Score 2 (NEWS2)

Here are two assessment tools that can be used together. The A-G assessment, based on the A-E guidance from the Resuscitation Council UK (2015a), is a systematic tool that you can use to do a top-to-toe assessment of the patient. The NEWS2 tool is a physiological assessment that – when combined with the A-G assessment – provides a complete holistic assessment of the patient (RCP, 2017). Remember to gain informed consent from the patient before you begin (for more information about informed consent, see Chapter 3).

1. Airway

If the patient has spoken to you during your initial assessment, you know that their airway is clear and patent (unobstructed). If, however, they are coughing, holding their throat or chest, flushed, and unable to speak to you in full sentences, they may have a partially or fully obstructed airway. This is very severe, and you need to act immediately. See the annotated further reading section at the end of the chapter for guidance on how to treat choking. If their airway is clear and patent, you can move on to the breathing assessment.

2. Breathing (NEWS2: respiratory rate and peripheral oxygen saturation percentage)

First, you need to complete a respiratory assessment. For 15 initial seconds, you need to observe and take note of any respiratory noises, use of accessory muscles, shallow or deep inhalation, unequal chest expansion, or irregular breathing rhythms. After this, you need to count how many breaths the patient has during one full minute (a breath in and out counts as one breath). In total, your respiratory assessment should take 1 minute and 15 seconds. A word of caution: do not be tempted to cut these times short and multiply up (e.g. counting how many breaths in 30 seconds and doubling the number). It is imperative that you complete a full 1 minute and 15 seconds assessment because if a patient is going to deteriorate, the first vital sign calculated as part of NEWS2 is the respiratory rate, or what you observe in the first 15 seconds. You may see alternative practices where you work, but you are accountable for your own practice.

Next you need to measure the peripheral oxygen saturation percentage (SpO_2). You need to place a clean saturation probe on one of the patient's fingers and leave it there for approximately 10 to 15 seconds. Remember to ensure that the patient has warm hands and is not wearing nail varnish, as this prevents the saturation probe from working (ask permission to remove the nail varnish, or as a last resort place the probe on a toe or the pinna – top – of the patient's ear). According to the Royal College of Physicians, the SpO_2 should be 96 per cent or greater (RCP, 2017). Check your local trust's policy because some trusts choose to adhere to the British Thoracic Society's guidance of 94–98 per cent (British Thoracic Society, 2017). If the patient's SpO_2 is less than their target percentage, they may need to have oxygen administered. Check your local trust's policy for guidance on target values, particularly for patients with chronic obstructive pulmonary disease (COPD), and at what percentage you need to start emergency oxygen therapy at 15 litres per minute via a non-rebreather mask.

Now that you have measured two NEWS2 vital signs, it is recommended that you correctly record them on the NEWS2 chart so that you do not forget them (see the annotated further reading section at the end of the chapter).

3. Circulation (NEWS2: blood pressure and pulse rate)

There are three things you need to measure in the circulation section of the A-G assessment: blood pressure, pulse assessment and target fluid balance. Many trusts use a machine to automatically calculate blood pressure. The NMC *Standards of Proficiency for Nursing Associates* state that you must be able to use a manual sphygmomanometer (sphyg for short) to measure a patient's blood pressure, so you will need to ensure that you remain competent using each method. For both machines and sphygs, make sure that you use the correct size of cuff for the patient you are caring for. Sphyg cuffs come in paediatric to extra-large sizes; see the manufacturer's guidance of the sphyg you are using to make sure that you size it correctly. Remember to record these measurements on the NEWS2 chart.

The patient's pulse rate may be displayed on the automatic blood pressure machine. However, this number does not inform you about the strength and regularity of the pulse; the only way to assess these is by doing a manual pulse assessment. Place three fingers on the radial pulse for 15 seconds to establish the strength and regularity of the pulse, then count the pulse rate for 60 seconds.

To calculate the target fluid balance for the patient, you need to know their age and weight. Use these values in the equations below to establish the target fluid input and output:

1. Input

    - Aged 59 years or younger: 35 ml × total weight (kg) = target fluid (ml) input in 24 hours
    - Aged 60 years or older: 30 ml × total weight (kg) = target fluid (ml) input in 24 hours

2. Output

    - All adult ages: 0.5 ml × total weight (kg) × 24 hours = total fluid (ml) output in 24 hours

3. Paediatric fluid balance

    - Infants and children need different amounts of fluid and excrete different amounts of fluid, depending on their age and weight. These values differ slightly between each trust and local authority, so make sure that you check your local trust's policy and/or guidance.

4. Dysfunction (NEWS2: level of responsiveness)

In the dysfunction stage (also known as disability), there are six assessments that you need to make, which are summarised below. First, you need to assess the patient's responsiveness using another acronym, 'ACVPU':

Alert

Confused

Voice

Pain

Unresponsive

If the patient is alert, they will be looking at you and **orientated** to the correct time, place and person (e.g. who you are). If they are talking to you but not orientated to time, place or person, they are confused. In the event that they do not engage in conversation, you need to check their response to your voice by giving them a simple command such as, 'Open your eyes.' If they do not carry out your

(Continued)

(Continued)

command, test their response to pain by squeezing their shoulder muscle (trapezium) with your thumb and fingers. This is the only way that anyone can assess a patient's response to pain – never attempt any others. Always remember 'squeeze the trapeze' when assessing response to pain. If the patient does not respond to any of the above, they are classed as unresponsive and you need to call for help from a nurse or doctor immediately. Remember to record your findings on the NEWS2 chart.

If the patient is diabetic or you observe hypoglycaemic (low blood sugar) or hyperglycaemic (high blood sugar) **signs** or **symptoms**, you need to measure their CBG level. See the annotated further reading section at the end of the chapter for more information on what is considered a safe CBG level.

If the patient is in pain, you need to assess this thoroughly. There are many pain assessment tools, but you could use the initialism 'PQRST' to help you:

*P*rovoke and *P*alliate

*Q*uality

*R*adiate

*S*everity

*T*ime

These are questions that you can ask the patient about their pain, such as 'What makes the pain worse?' (provoke) and 'What makes the pain better?' (palliate). Ask the patient to describe what their pain feels like (quality). Do not ask leading questions here, but rather open questions, such as 'Describe to me what your pain feels like.' The next question might be 'Does your pain spread anywhere?' (radiate). You need to measure how bad the pain is, so you might ask, 'On a scale of zero to three, zero being no pain at all and three being the worst pain you have ever experienced, where would you rate your pain?' The 0–3 scale aligns with the World Health Organization's pain scale ladder, which is particularly useful for patients living with cancer (WHO, 2019); however, your trust may use a 0–10 pain scale, so remember to check their policy.

Pain is a common symptom of constipation, which many patients suffer from across their lifespan. You can use the Bristol stool chart, adapted by the Central and North West London NHS Foundation Trust (2015), to help you identify what type of stool the patient last had.

The medications the patient is taking may be affecting their bowels, so you need to ask questions such as:

1. What medications have you been prescribed?
2. Which medications have you continued to take?
3. Are you taking any over-the-counter or homeopathic medication?
4. Do you use any recreational drugs?

Remember to escalate these findings to the prescriber, pharmacist or registered nurse you are working with.

Lastly, you need to assess how mobile the patient is and if this has recently changed. Remember to ask if they have a fear of falling or have had a fall in the last six months (for guidance on caring for patients at risk of falling, see the annotated further reading section at the end of the chapter).

5. Exposure (NEWS2: temperature)

The last vital sign to measure in the A-G assessment is the patient's temperature. According to NEWS2, the patient's temperature should be between 36.1 and 38.0 °C (RCP, 2017). A higher temperature than this is known as **hyperthermia** and a lower temperature is known as **hypothermia**.

The last few things to assess are the integrity of the patient's skin (look for pressure sores, wounds, rashes or discolouration), checking if they have any allergies (you could do this during your initial assessment when first meeting the patient), asking if they have been eating normally for them or if there have been any changes, and lastly any other tests or investigations that the patient may need (e.g. an X-ray for a broken wrist). Remember to objectively record the findings in the patient's care plan or assessment record.

6. Family and friends

Lastly, you need to complete a quick social care assessment. Identify who the patient's next of kin or main point of contact is and offer to contact them (if the patient would like you to). If appropriate, discuss with the patient if they have an existing package of social care at home or if they think they need one. This will inform the process of discharge planning.

7. Goals

You are now at the end of your A-G assessment. It is time to calculate the total NEWS2 score (for more information on using this tool, see the annotated further reading section at the end of the chapter) and identify the patient's goals. Each goal needs to be recorded in the patient's care plan, which you will read about later in this chapter, and each goal needs to meet the following requirements:

*S*pecific

*M*easurable

*A*chievable

*R*ealistic

*T*imely

You can see that the first letter of each requirement spells 'SMART'. Remembering this acronym and using it as a checklist when identifying the patient's goals will ensure that you are adhering to the principles of person-centred care.

Once you have completed your A-D and A-G assessments, you may need to hand over the pateint's care to someone else or escalate their condition because they are about to clinically or psychologically deteriorate. There is one more acronym, 'SBAR', which is very useful for keeping your handover or escalation succinct, as well as ensuring that you communicate effectively.

Understanding the theory: situation, background, assessment, recommendation (SBAR)

One of your aims as a nursing associate when caring for a patient is to recognise if a patient is about to deteriorate, or to react promptly if they have already started to become acutely unwell.

(Continued)

(Continued)

The deterioration may be a new acute illness or an **exacerbation** of a long-term condition. In either scenario, you will complete A-D and A-G assessments. Linking back to the nursing process, you have now completed the assessment, planning and nursing diagnosis stages. You now need to implement your plan, which for any deteriorating patient is to escalate to a senior member of nursing or medical staff (this may be the ambulance service, if you are working in the community).

In the heat of the moment, your stress levels are likely to be raised, and it is very easy to rush your communication in this situation. Using a systematic tool such as 'SBAR' will support you to communicate effectively and efficiently, proven by Müller et al.'s (2018) **systematic review**, which investigated the impact of using 'SBAR' to communicate among healthcare staff. The information below is based on Table 1 in Müller et al. (2018, p2).

1. Situation

Whether you are speaking on the phone or in person, if your colleague does not know you, make sure that you introduce yourself using the principles of #hellomynameis. Identify which patient you are escalating or handing over by stating their name. Now state the patient's predominant concern in a short sentence. It may sound something like, 'Mrs Gibson is having severe abdominal pain.' Keeping this sentence short will capture your colleague's attention; you need them to hear about the important information you have just gathered during your assessment.

2. Background

Next your colleague needs to know the patient's background. You only need to state the relevant past medical history and recent events that led to the current situation. Similarly, keep this section short so your key message does not get lost in surplus information. You may say something like, 'Mrs Gibson was brought to A&E because of the pain and she has not urinated for 10 to 12 hours. Her relevant past medical history is that she has insulin-dependent Type 2 diabetes.'

3. Assessment

Now is the time to share the important information you have gathered during your A-D and A-G assessments. Just as before, only share relevant information. In other words, you do not need to tell your colleague every vital sign that you have recorded on the NEWS2 chart. Simply state the overall NEWS2 score and which vital signs are a concern. For example, you might say, 'Mrs Gibson's respiratory rate is 22 breaths per minute, her pulse rate is 140 beats per minute, and her temperature is 38.5 °C. This makes the overall NEWS2 score 6. Her blood pressure does not score on NEWS2 because it is 180/90 mmHg. However, because she is diabetic, her target systolic blood pressure should be 135 mmHg or lower, so she is **hypertensive** too.'

4. Recommendation

If you have a clinical impression, you can say this now. You might state, 'I think she has urinary sepsis.' It is equally acceptable to say that you are not sure what is wrong with the patient you are caring for; saying that you do not know what is wrong will further encourage your colleague to help you. You now need to ask your colleague to come with you to see that patient. State a realistic time frame of when you think your colleague needs to see the patient, such as, 'I would like you to see the patient within the next 30 minutes, please.' If the patient is critically unwell like Mrs Gibson, you may need to be professionally assertive and say, 'I would like you to come with me now to see Mrs Gibson, please, because I am very concerned.' Before you end the conversation, ask your colleague, 'Is there anything more I can do now?'

So far in this chapter, you have read about four tools you can use in clinical practice that can help you care for patients with acute or long-term conditions. In relation to the implementation stage of the nursing process, read Annexe B of the *Standards of Proficiency for Nursing Associates* for a list of procedures within your scope of practice (NMC, 2018a). Next you will read about providing person-centred care across the lifespan and within the context of the four fields nursing.

Person-centred care across the lifespan

It has been emphasised many times in this book so far that the differences between people are something to celebrate, but there is one thing that unites everyone: we all experience the same stages of the lifespan. You will read about each stage of the lifespan throughout the next sections of this chapter (adapted from Armstrong, 2019). Reading the following box will provide you with an overview of the human lifespan.

Understanding the theory: the human lifespan

Pregnancy

The term of pregnancy is approximately nine months from conception to birth. The care of pregnant women is an interesting topic, and there are many textbooks to inform your knowledge. A salient point here is that your duty of care is to the woman, first and foremost. This poses an ethical debate; you could have a discussion about the laws surrounding the care of pregnant women with your supervisor or senior colleague if you are going to work in a maternity environment. Remember not to identify a pregnant woman as a patient – it is perfectly healthy to be pregnant.

Birth

Your role as a nursing associate in relation to the birth of a child is to support the MDT (particularly the midwife), as well as the mother and her family. Your A-D and A-G assessment skills will be vitally important here, including your skills at measuring vital signs using NEWS2. If a birth is complex, the child will be transferred to a paediatric unit after birth, whereas the mother will be cared for in an adult nursing environment. If at all possible, mother and baby will be kept in the same clinical environment to help with bonding.

Infancy

The age of an infant is approximately 0–3 years, but this age range may differ depending on what literature you read. One of the most important care needs of an infant is to monitor their growth and development. Each local trust will have a policy on how this is measured, but every tool is a holistic assessment of growth and development. If you have been signed off as competent in your trust to complete these assessments, you are likely to be working in the community assisting a home visiting team; however, you could be working in an inpatient paediatric assessment unit.

(Continued)

(Continued)

Childhood

Childhood is from approximately the age of 3 until puberty. These are pertinent developmental years, both physically and psychologically. Great Ormond Street Hospital in London is the national hospital for the specialised care of children. Visit their website for more information about the acute and long-term conditions that they specialise in: **www.gosh.nhs.uk**

Adolescence

Another phrase for adolescence is 'teenage years'. It is difficult to put an exact age on when puberty begins because each child is different. The physical health of adolescence has been well documented; however, historically, the mental health of adolescence was overlooked. Thankfully, in modern practice, adolescent mental health is taken more seriously.

Early adulthood

Early adulthood can be when many young people gain their first independence from their parents or guardians, but never presume that this is the case. Patient education during this stage of the lifespan is very important, particularly on how to maintain health and wellbeing.

Midlife

The importance of patient education continues in midlife. Maintaining a healthy work–life balance is significant for patients' physical and psychological health. Due to poor lifestyle choices, this is the stage of life when some long-term conditions may start to present themselves. Diabetes was discussed earlier in this chapter; people who are overweight and aged 40 years or older are at high risk of gaining Type 2 diabetes.

Late adulthood

It is during this stage of the lifespan that people may choose to retire. As patients become older, particularly in the modern age when we are living longer, multiple long-term conditions may be diagnosed. With advances in healthcare, many people can continue to live a very active and healthy life in late adulthood.

Elderly

People who are elderly (approximately 80 years of age or older) can similarly be very healthy and active if they maintain positive lifestyle choices and good health and wellbeing habits. In some cases, however, people living with many co-morbidities may have complex care needs to manage their physical and psychological health.

End of life

End of life care is defined as the last 12 months of a patient's life. This can be difficult to determine, and hence end of life care is a clinical specialism. You may hear the term '**palliative care**' in reference to caring for someone who is dying, although palliative care is defined as managing a long-term condition. End of life care can last for more than six months, so it is a long-term condition, but remember that the term 'palliative care' may be in reference to another long-term condition.

Now that you have read about the stages of the lifespan and have had some suggestions of what care a patient may need at each stage, complete Activity 2.3 to put your learning into context.

Activity 2.3   Reflection

The next time you are in clinical practice, discuss with your supervisor or line manager which stage of the lifespan a patient may be in. Do not use their age as an indicator; the more important things to observe here are their care needs. By being able to identify the patient's care needs, you will more accurately and confidently be able to provide person-centred care.

As this activity is based on your own reflection, there is no outline answer provided at the end of the chapter.

The different needs that patients have at each stage of their lifespan can be met within the context of the four fields of nursing. As a nursing associate, you are a generalist practitioner, so your clinical knowledge and skills will transcend all four fields of nursing. If in practice, however, you need to get some more advice about how to care for a patient with a particular need, speak to a practitioner that specialises in one of these fields. By doing this, you are demonstrating that you are working within your scope of practice and linking other members of the MDT together to provide person-centred care for the patient in your care.

Person-centred care in the four fields of nursing

The nursing profession is currently separated into four specialised fields: adult, paediatric, mental health and learning disability. The rationale behind having four specialisms is that since nursing students' education is so in depth, they choose to study a course that focuses on one of the four fields of nursing. Having a deeper understanding of one field of nursing enables practitioners to strengthen their knowledge and skills, thus better understanding patients' needs. There are some generic topics to study that are applicable to all four fields of nursing; however, the remainder of undergraduate nurses' training is bespoke to their chosen field of nursing.

Although nurses have a specialism, every nurse must adhere to *The Code* (NMC, 2018b), just like nursing associates. Fundamentally, all nurses are expected to be competent at providing basic nursing care. Within their respective specialisms, however, nurses will have more specific knowledge and skills that they can use to care for patients with particular needs. For example, all nurses have a basic understanding of how to communicate with someone that is living with depression. A mental health nurse, however, has significantly more knowledge and understanding about how to complete a mental health assessment for someone living with depression, as well as what care they may need.

How does this relate to you as a nursing associate? Nurses have a specific scope of practice within their chosen field of nursing. Nursing Associates are, as previously mentioned, generalist practitioners. This does not mean that nursing associates are miniature nurses. This is impossible because you are a different practitioner, with your own professional registration; in other words, you are not registered with the NMC as a 'miniature nurse'. Nursing associates' scope of practice is to provide fundamental care from not just one field of nursing, but all four.

Your training as a nursing associate gives you exposure to all four fields of nursing, both academically and in clinical practice. (However, your learning does not stop at the end of your apprenticeship. To find out more about how to keep up to date with the future of providing person-centred care, see Chapter 8.) As a fully qualified and registered nursing associate, you will be able to use your knowledge and experience to support nurses and the MDT while working independently to meet the needs of the patients in your care. You must always work within your scope of practice, so make sure that you read and continually familiarise yourself with the *Standards of Proficiency for Nursing Associates* (NMC, 2018a).

Person-centred care plans

Care plans are formal records of a patient's previous assessments and treatments, as well as instructions on what their current care needs are. Care plans are needed as a communication tool between practitioners and support workers in the MDT. A care plan can be used to evidentially measure if the patient is getting better or deteriorating, as well as determining if their condition remains the same. A care plan is also a legal record of what care has been provided for the patient by the healthcare service; this is important to protect the safety of the patient, as well as the professionals looking after them. Although nursing associates do not write care plans, it is within your scope of practice to evaluate them, as well as suggesting changes or updates to the registered nurse that you are working alongside. You must consider all documentation in your clinical practice to be legal documents. Accurate and evidence-based record-keeping is hence considered a vital skill for a nursing associate. In Chapter 5, we will discuss inclusivity in person-centred care. A care plan is bespoke to an individual patient, so your ability to be inclusive when reading and evaluating care plans is paramount to maintaining person-centred care. The Royal College of Nursing (RCN) has published guidance on the principles of good record-keeping, which is freely available for you to download (RCN, 2017). Use this guidance to complete Activity 2.4.

Activity 2.4   Reflection

For this activity, you can use any word-processing software, your email account, or a pen and notebook. To practise objective record-keeping, write down the following:

1. *A record of what happened today.* This record could be about your day at university, in clinical practice, or what you did on a day off. You need to ensure that you are writing objectively (i.e. only write down the facts of what happened). You may wish to record your feelings or interpretations in a separate paragraph, but make sure to keep the first paragraph focused on facts. Remember to maintain confidentiality if you are writing about clinical practice.
2. *A plan of what you would like to achieve tomorrow.* Your plan for tomorrow should be listed in order of priority, and each point must meet all components of a SMART goal (see earlier in this chapter). Make sure that you consider what a realistic list of targets would be for tomorrow; achieving three goals in total is much more satisfying than achieving three goals out of ten that you have written down.

You could focus this activity on your studying to help you maintain focus, or you could use it as a reflective tool to help you continue to learn from clinical practice. This activity can be a single exercise, or you may choose to continue it over an extended period of time if you find it a useful exercise.

As this activity is based on your own reflection, there is no outline answer provided at the end of the chapter.

A key question to ask yourself about any of your record-keeping in clinical practice is, 'Does my care plan evaluation remain focused on providing person-centred care?' If the answer is yes, then you have written a good care plan. Linking back to the nursing process at the beginning of the chapter, the next stage after planning is to implement care. For this stage, nursing associates must have very good interpersonal skills and communication techniques.

Interpersonal skills and communication techniques for person-centred care

In the chapter so far, you may have recognised that the patients you care for each have their own backgrounds, conditions and healthcare needs. As a result, you need to be able to frequently adapt and develop your interpersonal skills and communication techniques to be able to efficiently build a rapport with patients. You need to earn their trust before you will be able to provide the best quality person-centred care. This requires extensive and consistent practice, but reading this section will point you in the right direction.

Being **interpersonal** in health and social care can be defined as establishing professional relationships between people, as well as using appropriate communication and building connections with them. To be interpersonal is significantly important for nursing associates because you need to earn patients' trust. Achieving this will encourage patients to feel relaxed, as well as being forthcoming about their acute and long-term conditions. When patients are relaxed enough to be honest about their health, you will be able to complete a thorough holistic assessment, as well as monitoring their health and evaluating the outcomes. From reading this chapter so far, it will be clear to you that a rigorous assessment is vital to ensure that patients' acute and long-term conditions are cared for appropriately.

So, how do you ensure that your practice is interpersonal? There is no rulebook on interpersonal skills, but it is likely that you already use them on a daily basis. Becoming more self-aware of them will enable you to enhance these skills in practice. According to Mind Tools (2019b), to have interpersonal skills requires **emotional intelligence**, as well as being able to recognise other people's emotions by their expressions, mannerisms and tone of voice. You are then able to adjust your communication with patients to build a connection with them. For example, if a patient appears upset but does not vocalise it, you can demonstrate empathy by acknowledging that they appear upset and asking if there is anything you can do for them. Once a patient starts to trust you, you need to consolidate this trust by using **active listening**. Actively listening means that you demonstrate your understanding of what a patient is telling you; repeating what they have said in your own words may do this, or you could simply state that you understand their point of view (providing you do understand!). If you are unsure what their key message is, show that you are trying to understand by saying something like, 'I am not sure what you mean; could you explain it in a different way?' With this in mind, you clearly need to have bespoke **communication** skills to be able to provide interpersonal person-centred care. Think carefully about how you are communicating and question if there is a more appropriate method.

You may need to use picture cards, ask the patient to write down what they are saying, or request an interpreter. Effective communication between patients and practitioners is imperative, similar to communication within the MDT.

As discussed earlier in the chapter, documentation and record-keeping is one communication technique that nursing associates need to be masters of. Remember that you are a link between all practitioners in the MDT; therefore, your documentation and record-keeping must be immaculate so that all of your colleagues can read the important information you have gathered about a patient. Professionals in the MDT, however, are not the only people you need to be able to communicate with. As discussed in Chapter 1, the NHS serves the public. Patients are considered the most important members of the MDT, because without them there is no NHS. In the annotated further reading section at the end of the chapter, there is suggested guidance for you on record-keeping.

Chapter summary

There is a lot of content in this chapter, which is representative of the knowledge required to understand person-centred care of acute and long-term conditions. As previously noted, reading this chapter provides you with the tools to use in clinical practice to care for patients with acute and long-term conditions. It is impossible to include intricate details on how to care for each acute and long-term condition, but you will now be able to recognise differences between the two, as well as what stage of the lifespan a patient is in. The nursing process is applicable to all acute and long-term conditions, so you can use this as a guide for providing person-centred care. Remember to practise using the assessment tools discussed in this chapter and seek feedback from your supervisor or line manager, as well as keeping yourself up to date with new developments in evidence-based practice and the interpersonal skills you need.

Activities: Brief outline answers

All of the activities in this chapter are based on your own reflection, so there are no outline answers.

Annotated further reading

Howatson-Jones, L., Standing, M. and Roberts, S. (2015) *Patient Assessment and Care Planning in Nursing*, 2nd edition. London: SAGE.

This book is succinct and written in a clear and concise style. Chapter 1 focuses on reason-centred assessment, which is relevant to your role as a nursing associate. However, this book has been written for nurses, so be mindful that some of the content is not within your scope of practice. If you are unsure about what is in your scope of practice, check the *Standards of Proficiency for Nursing Associates* (NMC, 2018a).

National Institute for Health and Care Excellence (NICE) (2013) *Falls in Older People: Assessing Risk and Prevention.* Available at: www.nice.org.uk/guidance/cg161

Falls are a very common cause of acute conditions. This NICE guidance provides information about which patients are at risk of falling, as well as what you can do to mitigate that risk.

National Institute for Health and Care Excellence (NICE) (2016) *Diabetes (Type 1 and Type 2) in Children and Young People.* Available at: www.nice.org.uk/guidance/ng18

National Institute for Health and Care Excellence (NICE) (2016) *Type 1 Diabetes in Adults.* Available at: www.nice.org.uk/guidance/ng17

National Institute for Health and Care Excellence (NICE) (2019) *Type 2 Diabetes in Adults.* Available at: www.nice.org.uk/guidance/ng28

Diabetes is a long-term condition with many categories to understand. These works provide you with a link to guidance on Type 1, Type 2 and paediatric diabetes diagnosis and management.

Resuscitation Council UK (2015) *Choking.* Available at: www.resus.org.uk/choking/

Read this guidance on choking to know the process of how to treat someone who has a partially or fully obstructed airway. You can find the adult and paediatric guidelines via this link.

Royal College of Nursing (RCN) (2017) *Record Keeping: The Facts.* Available at: www.rcn.org.uk/professional-development/publications/pub-006051

You can use this fact sheet about documentation and record-keeping to self-asses the standard of your documentation. The RCN has published additional articles about other principles of documentation, which you can search for on its website.

Tait, D., James, J., Williams, C. and Barton, D. (2016) *Acute and Critical Care in Adult Nursing,* 2nd edition. London: SAGE.

This is another well-written book that is helpfully compartmentalised into different types of acute conditions that patients may experience, such as breathlessness, pain and psychological shock. This book is also written primarily for nurses, so make sure to read the sections relevant to nursing associates.

Useful websites

American Institute for Learning and Human Development – The 12 Stages of Life: www.institute4learning.com/resources/articles/the-12-stages-of-life/

This web page provides more information about Armstrong's (2019) work on the stages of the lifespan.

Mind Tools: www.mindtools.com

Visit this website for more information on interpersonal skills and communication techniques.

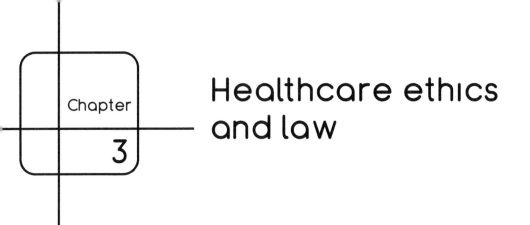

Healthcare ethics and law

Chapter 3

Chapter aims

After reading this chapter, you will be able to:

- identify key legislation relating to your role as a nursing associate;
- identify ethical principles that affect person-centred care;
- recognise the importance of safeguarding;
- reflect on learning from legal and ethical case studies.

Introduction

The Code (NMC, 2018b) and the *Standards of Proficiency for Nursing Associates* (NMC, 2018a) were introduced in Chapter 1. These documents are a guide for you to provide person-centred care for patients. Reading and applying evidence in acute and long-term care, as discussed in Chapter 2, is equally as important for person-centred care. However, law and ethics are two topics that are similarly fundamental to keeping patients safe. Law and ethics are very broad subjects, and, as a nursing associate, you need to be familiar with relevant legislation and ethical principles to ensure that your practice is safe. In this chapter, key legislation will be discussed, and you will be able to identify how it relates to clinical practice. Law, however, is only one side of the coin. Learning about the principles of ethics will enable you to think about practice-based case studies in alternative ways and reflect on your own person-centred care. There may not be an easy or comfortable answer to some situations in practice, so you can use your learning from ethical case studies in this chapter to support your decision-making. Ethics and law may seem like opposite ends of a spectrum, but by the end of this chapter you will see how interdependent they are.

Introduction to law

Laws are the rules of the UK that everyone must abide by, also known as pieces of legislation (UK Parliament, 2019). Laws are created by Parliament, which is made up of the House of Commons, the House of Lords and the sovereign (Her Majesty The Queen). The House of Commons consists of 650 democratically elected Members of Parliament (MPs), whereas the House of Lords contains approximately 800 members who are appointed by the sovereign on advice from the Prime Minister or who have a hereditary entitlement. To begin the process of creating a law, members of the House of Commons or the House of Lords propose a Bill. A Bill can be described as a new, draft law or a suggested amendment to an existing law. Bills are passed between both Houses of Parliament so that the content can be debated. However, if a Bill is passed by the House of Commons in two consecutive years or the Bill is about tax and/or public expenses, it does not need to be sent to the House of Lords. Once both Houses of Parliament agree, a Bill is upgraded to an Act of Parliament (also known as primary legislation) and sent to the sovereign for royal assent (approval).

An Act of Parliament contains the basic information of a new law or amendment to an existing law. The government, the political party – or coalition of parties – with the most members in the House of Commons, then begins to refine the content of an Act of Parliament and prepare for it to be implemented. The government has the responsibility to implement the law correctly within a specific time frame. Some Acts of Parliament are more urgent than others, so each Act of Parliament is enforced within different periods of time. Once the Act of Parliament has been fully enforced, it is known as law. There is a helpful video available on the UK Parliament's website, which can be found in the annotated further reading section at the end of the chapter.

You now know the process of how a law is created, but what types of laws are there? The short answer is that there are many, but not all of them are related to health and social care. The following box illustrates the different types of law, as well as a short explanation of what they focus on. The laws listed here apply to England and Wales only; Northern Ireland and Scotland have their own legal systems and classes of law. Next in this chapter, specific laws are focused on, as well as how they relate to your practice.

> # Understanding the theory: classes of English and Welsh law
>
> There are many classes of law, and as a nursing associate on a professional register you need to be able to identify relevant laws, understand the content, and ensure that your clinical practice is compliant. Below is a list of some classes of English and Welsh laws that you need to have knowledge of. If you work in a different country, you will need to check their laws as there will be differences:
>
> - *Statutory law*: Also known as legislation, this is a law that has been enacted by the procedure described in the 'Introduction to law' section of this chapter.
> - *Criminal law*: A law that is in place to prosecute criminals who have been proven guilty of committing an offence.
> - *Case law*: A law that has been established following a legal case, which has now become legislation.
>
> Every individual law will be in a class of law. You do not need to memorise the classes of law, but you will need to be able to read and understand relevant legislation.

As you have read, there are many types of law that focus on different subjects. There are a number of laws that apply to healthcare and your practice as a nursing associate. The predominant legislation that empowers the NMC to be a governing body is the Nursing and Midwifery Order 2001. You can find out more about the NMC's legal framework on its website (NMC, 2019). Amendments have been made recently to include nursing associates, so the NMC is also your governing body and regulator. The Nursing and Midwifery Order 2001 is important to be aware of, but there are other laws that are related more closely to your clinical practice. You therefore need to be able to search for legislation online, read it, and understand how to apply it to your clinical practice to ensure that you are keeping yourself and patients safe. Complete Activity 3.1 to practise searching for some laws.

Activity 3.1   Critical thinking

Search the website **www.legislation.gov.uk** for a law that you think may be relevant to you as a nursing associate. Read the summary, as well as perhaps a lengthier section, and write down another summary of the law in your own words using no more than 200 words (one paragraph). Write your summary as if you were going to explain the content of the law you have read to another nursing associate who has not read that law before. By doing this, you will be consolidating your own understanding of a law and – if you share your summary – helping a colleague to understand it too.

(Continued)

(Continued)

If you are ever in any doubt about the meaning of a law (or any policy, guidance or document), you should discuss this with your supervisor or line manager before taking any action. The Royal College of Nursing has useful information and offers free legal advice, if you are a member (RCN, 2020a).

As this activity is based on your own reflection, there is no outline answer provided at the end of the chapter.

Activity 3.1 encourages you to interact with a law by reading the original text and summarising it in your own words. This is a useful exercise to help you to understand law and succinctly explain how it applies to your practice. You could also share your written summary with a colleague to get feedback on your academic writing, as well as supporting them in understanding law. There are some key laws that you need to be familiar with, which are explored in the next section.

Key health and social care laws

This section of the chapter has been written in smaller paragraphs to provide you with a succinct summary of key health and social care laws. It is important to note that you cannot rely on this section to inform you enough to have a complete understanding of key health and social care laws. Remember that newly created laws may override existing laws and current laws can be amended. The aim of this section is to provide you with a summary of some key laws that you can read before reading the law itself. This section will also serve as a revision aide of the topics of key health and social care laws, but to reiterate: laws are periodically updated, so you must ensure that you check the original document for amendments – changes are usually summarised at the beginning of a law. The laws discussed in this section are:

- Health and Social Care Act 2012;
- Equality Act 2010;
- Mental Capacity Act 2005.

The Health and Social Care Act 2012 was the biggest reform of the NHS since 1948. A notable change was the legal obligation for NHS organisations to actively reduce **health inequality** across the country, particularly for the Department of Health (since renamed to Department of Health and Social Care, DHSC), Public Health England (PHE), NHS England, and clinical commissioning groups (CCGs) (King's Fund, 2016). CCGs were given control of budgets to fund local services, the theory being that local groups would have a contextual understanding of local services' needs. In 2016, the King's Fund wrote a review of the impact of the Health and Social Care Act 2012 and submitted it to the House of Commons Health Committee, which can be found in the annotated further reading section at the end of the chapter. The NHS will inevitably continue to change year on year. This change is guided by the strategic *NHS Long Term Plan* document (NHS Long Term Plan, 2019). For more information on how to keep yourself up to date with an ever-changing NHS, see Chapter 8. Before you read on, complete Activity 3.2 to deepen your understanding of the Health and Social Care Act 2012.

Activity 3.2   Critical thinking

The Health and Social Care Act 2012 is a pivotal moment in the recent history of the NHS, defining the way the NHS operates as an organisation. The information is very high level (to be generalisable), and as a nursing associate you need to be able to identify how this key piece of legislation applies to your practice. Read the overview of the Health and Social Care Act 2012 fact sheets (GOV.UK, 2012) and identify where the content correlates with the *Standards of Proficiency for Nursing Associates* (NMC, 2018a). You can find the weblink to the Health and Social Care Act 2012 fact sheets in the annotated further reading section at the end of the chapter. Discuss your thoughts with your supervisor or line manager.

An outline answer is provided at the end of the chapter.

The Health and Social Care Act 2012 has had a huge influence of the way the NHS is structured at large, as wel as having an indirect impact on your clinical practice. The budgets for the services you work in are decided by CCGs, and it is the Health and Social Care Act 2012 that empowers CCGs to do this. Another key law that has a direct impact on your clinical practice is the Mental Capacity Act 2005. The Mental Capacity Act was originally published in 2005, although the current version is the Mental Capacity (Amendment) Act 2019. The purpose of the Mental Capacity (Amendment) Act 2019 is to protect people who are not safe to make decisions about their care, as well as empowering them to make decisions supported by a nominated **lasting power of attorney** (NHS, 2018b). In other words, the Mental Capacity (Amendment) Act 2019 legally obligates a designated, trustworthy person (usually a family member or friend) to ensure that the patient makes safe decisions about their care. An example from clinical practice would be a patient living with advanced dementia having a close family member, friend or carer be their lasting power of attorney. This person would make decisions on behalf of the patient, with their best interests in mind. There are many grey areas regarding mental capacity, some of which are discussed later in this chapter. Complete Activity 3.3 before you read on.

Activity 3.3   Evidence-based practice and research

The Mental Capacity (Amendment) Act 2019 protects people who need support in making decisions for themselves about their care. There are lots of conditions and situations where someone needs protecting under the Mental Capacity (Amendment) Act 2019. Search online, using valid and reliable websites, for examples of when the Mental Capacity (Amendment) Act 2019 is needed to protect someone – the NHS website is an ideal website to visit. There are many situations where the Mental Capacity (Amendment) Act 2019 may need to be used in clinical practice. Later in this chapter, some case studies explore how the Mental Capacity (Amendment) Act 2019 has protected people and ensured that they received person-centred care.

An outline answer is provided at the end of the chapter.

Completing Activity 3.3 will illustrate to you that there are many different patient conditions and situations where they require protection under the Mental Capacity (Amendment) Act 2019. However, this is not the only law that protects people. The Equality Act 2010 legally supports and safeguards people who have one of nine protected characteristics from discrimination. The nine protected characteristics are:

- age;
- disability;
- gender reassignment;
- marriage and civil partnership;
- pregnancy and maternity;
- race;
- religion or belief;
- sex;
- sexual orientation.

There was legislation to protect people from discrimination before this law; however, it was broken into different Acts of Parliament that were difficult to navigate. The passing of the Equality Act 2010 provided one law that includes all protected characteristics, and thus the legislation is much easier to understand (GOV.UK, 2015). The Equality Act 2010 includes both negative and positive discrimination. Negative discrimination is deliberately harming someone, physically or psychologically, because of their protected characteristic(s), whereas positive discrimination is the unfair favouritism of a person with a protected characteristic. As you can see, the peripheries of the Equality Act 2010 are not distinct; the law is enforced on the basis of context and situation. The Equality Act 2010 has many links with the principles of ethics, which you can read about in the next section of this chapter. Before you do this, complete Activity 3.4 to increase your confidence and understanding of the Equality Act 2010.

Activity 3.4   Critical thinking

The Equality Act 2010 protects people from positive or negative discrimination of one or more of the nine protected characteristics a person may have. This law is very likely to apply to many, if not all, of the patients for whom you care. The Equality Act 2010 affects your clinical practice very frequently, perhaps every day. As a nursing associate, you need to be able to recognise if someone has a protected characteristic and is supported appropriately. Moreover, you need to be able to identify if a patient is being positively or negatively discriminated against. Make a list of hypothetical situations where someone may be being positively or negatively discriminated against due to one or more protected characteristics. Discuss these with your supervisor or line manager the next time you have a meeting with them.

If you do think that a patient, family member or friend is being discriminated against, you must act swiftly, but with caution – rash action may make the situation worse. Your course of action must be to ensure that the patient is safe, as well as immediately informing your supervisor or line manager to raise a concern. This links with safeguarding, which will be discussed later in this chapter.

As this activity is based on your own reflection, there is no outline answer provided at the end of the chapter.

The laws discussed in this chapter are not the only laws you need to understand. Furthermore, laws are frequently updated or established, so you need to ensure that your awareness of the law is current. With this in mind, it is imperative that you keep up to date with amendments to current laws, as well as the publication of new laws, to ensure that your clinical practice is legally compliant. Completing Activity 3.5 will help you to keep your knowledge of law up to date, before moving on to read about the principles of ethics and how they affect your ability to provide person-centred care.

Activity 3.5   Evidence-based practice and research

The website **www.gov.uk** is where the government publishes new and amended laws. They are freely available for you to read, download and share with colleagues. Keeping yourself updated can be very time-consuming if you have to keep checking the website to read publications; however, this activity will save you some time. When you go to the website, you can create email alerts. You can choose to have alerts from any government department, including the Department of Health and Social Care, as well as how often you receive email updates and which email address the updates are sent to. To ensure that you are updated regularly with changes to the law, set up an email alert to always be notified of any changes. You can find a link to the web page of the Department of Health and Social Care in the annotated further reading section at the end of the chapter.

As this activity is based on your own reflection, there is no outline answer provided at the end of the chapter.

You have now read a brief introduction to law and learned how it should be applied to your clinical practice at all times. Remember to always ensure that you keep up to date with changes to existing laws and new laws being created. As mentioned at the beginning of the chapter, the subject of ethics is very closely associated with law. Similarly, there are many principles of ethics (also known as ethical frameworks or models), and you need to have an understanding of them to ensure that your practice upholds the principles of person-centred care.

Ethics

Within the context of nursing associates and healthcare, ethics is about recognising what moral propositions you consider important and analysing how they affect your actions in different situations. In other words, ethics focuses on what you think is right or wrong in a particular scenario and analyses why you have this opinion (Ashcroft et al., 2007). Ethics applies to everyone in everyday life. Think about whether you prefer giving money to a homeless person or a charity for homeless people. This scenario may cause you to consider how much of a positive impact your donation may have for the homeless community. Making this decision at home is relatively straightforward because you are in a comfortable environment. However, would you make the same decision if a homeless person, who was crying, held out their hand and asked for any spare change?

Reflecting on your ethical principles (what you consider to be right or wrong) increases your self-awareness and can furthermore help you to make an informed decision when you are in an ethical dilemma. It is important to note, however, that your ethical principles may differ in comparison with your family, friends or colleagues; their ethical principles could be the polar opposite to yours. In any situation where there are differences, there is a need to be curious and understand alternative points of view. Unfortunately, history highlights many situations where people have chosen not to understand, which has catalysed fear, dislike or even violence. It is therefore important for you to be aware of your ethical principles, as well as how they connect with or differ from others, which this section of the chapter will explore.

As previously mentioned, ethics is a broad topic with many different ethical theories and frameworks. But how does ethics apply to your role as a nursing associate, and does it support you in providing person-centred care? According to Ashcroft et al. (2007), there are three subtypes of ethics that apply to healthcare: healthcare ethics, medical ethics and biomedical ethics. Medical ethics and biomedical ethics are more closely associated to medical practice, in comparison to nursing or nursing associate practice. Healthcare ethics focuses on ethical situations regarding the provision of holistic care; therefore, it is the type of ethics that is most relevant to you as a nursing associate. Activity 3.6 asks you to think about how your moral principles affect your clinical practice.

Activity 3.6   Reflection

Healthcare ethics is to do with ethical situations that you may come across when providing person-centred care. As discussed at the beginning of this section, your ethics is personal to you and ultimately determines how you will act in ethically sensitive situations. It is important to have self-awareness of your morals because this enables you to have self-awareness of how you choose to act. For this activity, make a list of characteristics that you identify as being good and a second list of characteristics that you identify as being bad (e.g. honesty, trustworthiness, vanity, empathy, disobedience, confidence). The good characteristics are what you value, whereas the bad characteristics may make you feel unhappy, angry or repulsed. This is important for you to be aware of in clinical practice because person-centred care and your professional body's code require you to care for patients with parity. Noting these morals will be useful later in this chapter, so keep them to hand.

As this activity is based on your own reflection, there is no outline answer provided at the end of the chapter.

Activity 3.6 will have encouraged you to reflect on your own morals and values, which inform your ethics. There are a number of ethical theories and frameworks that are helpful in explaining how what we have discussed so far affects your clinical practice. There are too many theories and frameworks to mention; however, some theories and frameworks are signposted in the next few sections. Do not feel that you can only use the theories and frameworks mentioned in this book. As part of your professional development, you may choose to read about alternative ethical models that can support your clinical practice. The following box provides a summary of two ethical models.

Understanding the theory: ethical theories

There are many ethical theories that can help you in evaluating an ethically sensitive situation that will inform your decision-making and actions. They can also support you in understanding why decisions or actions by other practitioners have been made. An example of an ethically sensitive situation is abortion. Many people raise valid points in support of or against this procedure, and ethical theories can help you to understand their perspectives. It is important to note that ethical theories do not tell you what to do in these situations, but guide your thought process. Always remember to follow *The Code* (NMC, 2018b) and the *Standards of Proficiency for Nursing Associates* (NMC, 2018a). There are two ethical theories that could inform your clinical practice:

- *Utilitarianism*: The principles of utilitarianism state that action should be taken if it benefits the majority of people. In some situations, such as creating a new law that protects people from harm, this may be a more moral choice. However, some situations are more challenging to debate. Assisted dying, for example, is a topic that many people have strong views about and raise valid points.
- *Deontology*: In contrast to the principles of utilitarianism, deontology always ethically determines the morality of the action itself, rather than the outcome of the action. A contextual example may be when an elderly patient with dementia is asking to see their parents (who died many years previously). The action of telling the patient that their parents have died (which risks the patient becoming upset) or agreeing with the patient that their parents will be arriving later (which makes the patient happy) is a deontological ethical debate.

There are many more ethical theories in addition to the two mentioned here. A brief explanation of how these two examples relate to clinical practice has been provided, but remember that alternative ethical theories may not be relevant to healthcare (or may even be inappropriate). Critical thinking is required to inform your decision about using an ethical theory to support your thought process in clinical practice.

The previous box has given you a summary of some ethical theories, but remember that there are many more. A seminal book about ethics is called *Principles of Biomedical Ethics* (Beauchamp and Childress, 2013). It is not a theory per se, like the ethical theories mentioned in the previous box, but it is a framework. Beauchamp and Childress (2013) developed four principles of biomedical ethics (i.e. ethics that applies to healthcare):

- respect for autonomy;
- non-maleficence;
- beneficence;
- justice.

The first principle applies to the patient's autonomy, which links to a requirement from *The Code* (NMC, 2018b). In other words, your role as a nursing associate requires you to empower the patient to have autonomy (where safe) to make their own informed decisions; you are putting them at the centre of their care. The second principle requires practitioners to avoid harming, injuring or hurting patients. Third, beneficence is closely associated with non-maleficence. Some healthcare interventions arguably cause harm to the patient; chemotherapy, for example, can have some very harmful side effects. However, the beneficence principle suggests that the benefits of chemotherapy outweigh the harm because the patient has a greater chance of survival. Lastly, the justice principle ensures that all care is provided to patients equally and fairly (i.e. providing person-centred care).

Now you have read a short introduction to ethics. Activity 3.7 contains a case study from clinical practice that exemplifies how to use an ethical framework to guide a clinical practitioner providing person-centred care. All of the people referred to in the case study have been given pseudonyms to maintain confidentiality.

Activity 3.7   Critical thinking and reflection

Thomas is a frail, elderly gentleman aged 96 years. He has many co-morbidities: hypertension, asthma, epilepsy and osteoarthritis. Thomas was admitted to hospital after a fall at home where he broke his hip. His surgery went well; however, during his stay in hospital, he has developed pneumonia and is feeling very low in mood. He has mental capacity but no longer wants to take his medication. His condition has deteriorated, and he needs antibiotics as well as his regular medications because he is at risk of developing sepsis and dying. His consultant explains this, and Thomas says he understands, but he does not want to take any more medication. There are no signs of him losing his mental capacity. He would like to sign a 'do not attempt resuscitation' (DNAR) form, also known as a 'do not resuscitate' (DNR) form. His children, Charles, Rachel and Jen, do not want him to sign a DNAR form. Discuss what ethical issues are presented in this case study with your supervisor or line manager. Identify which ethical theories or frameworks can be applied to Thomas' case. A suggested answer is available at the end of this chapter, but remember, each situation is different, so your experience in clinical practice is likely to differ.

An outline answer is provided at the end of the chapter, but remember that each situation is different, so your experience in clinical practice is likely to differ.

Activity 3.7 provided a contextual example of how the principles of ethics linked with clinical practice. The case study is a demonstration of how an ethical framework can be used to guide you when managing an ethical situation in clinical practice. It is important to emphasise that ethical frameworks do not instruct you on what to do, but rather provide direction and guidance. Remember the *The Code* (NMC, 2018b) is another document to support you in how to provide person-centred care, and your supervisor or line manager will be able to discuss your thoughts before acting. Another situation where you will need to have an immediate discussion with your supervisor or line manager is when there is a patient safeguarding concern.

Safeguarding

Safeguarding is a process within a hospital trust or healthcare service that protects vulnerable people or children from being abused. There are many different types of abuse, including but not limited to physical, emotional, sexual or online abuse (NSPCC, 2020). The healthcare service that you are an apprentice with or work for will provide you with safeguarding training, which will include how to identify a safeguarding concern and the necessary steps to ensure patient safety. Each hospital or healthcare service will have a slightly different policy, so they cannot all be mentioned in this book. However, an imperative point is that if you think a patient is at risk of or currently being abused in any way, immediately inform your supervisor or line manager in private. They will guide you regarding what needs to happen next.

Safeguarding is a very important part of your practice as a nursing associate. You spend a lot of time with patients; hence, it is likely that you will be one of the first practitioners to notice a safeguarding concern. It cannot be emphasised enough that you must know and understand the safeguarding policy of where you are working and be able to apply it in clinical practice from memory. Keep this knowledge up to date by rereading the policy and checking for any updates. The principles of ethics that have been discussed in this chapter provide another source of guidance that you can discuss with your line manager. Your documentation, particularly in relation to safeguarding, will be very significant. In addition to the self-assessment fact sheet listed in the annotated further reading section at the end of Chapter 2, you can also ask yourself, 'Would I be able to read my documentation in ten years' time and remember exactly what happened?' If the answer to this question is 'yes', then your documentation is detailed and clear enough. Remember to write concisely and objectively.

You have now read about law and ethics. However, in clinical practice, it is very likely that you will need to combine your knowledge of law and ethics to make a decision in the best interests of a patient while providing person-centred care. Activity 3.8 is another case study on how a law to protect young people is upheld, but an ethical principle guides the practitioner in making a person-centred decision.

Activity 3.8   Critical thinking

Victoria is a 13-year-old girl who has arranged to see her GP on her own. Victoria wants to ask for contraception but she does not want her family to know. The GP gives her advice about contraception. A few days later, Victoria's mother finds out what has happened and is furious with the GP, and lodges a formal complaint. Discuss this case study with your supervisor or line manager:

1. What laws relate to this case study?
2. Which ethical theories or frameworks relate to this case study?
3. Is there a safeguarding concern?

An outline answer is provided at the end of the chapter, but remember that each situation is different, so your experience in clinical practice is likely to differ.

The above case study is true; you can read about Victoria's story on the CQC's website (CQC, 2018). This case went to court, and as a result there is now 'Gillick competence' (named after Victoria's last name). A child aged 17 years or younger cannot normally give consent without a parent or guardian's permission, although in some situations 16- or 17-year-old children can make some decisions without their parents or guardians. However, if the child is deemed to be Gillick-competent, they are able to give consent. Similar to adults, informed consent must be given before any decision can be made about the child's care. The components of informed consent are:

*   the provision of sufficient information (good and bad);
*   the patient must be competent and understand all the information you have provided;
*   there must be no influence of bias on the patient from anyone;
*   the patient must have the power to withdraw their consent at any time.

Victoria's case raises some legal and ethical debates, and you may have very strong views about what is right or wrong in this situation. Remember that the law is in place to keep you and patients safe, and ethical theories and frameworks are there to help you understand rationale and actions, as well as understanding different perspectives.

Chapter summary

This chapter provides you with an overview of legislation and ethical philosophies that are relevant to you as a nursing associate. Remember that laws and ethics are periodically updated, so it is imperative that you keep your knowledge of law and ethics up to date, and thus keep your practice safe. The key legislation discussed in this chapter can be applied to most areas of practice, but always remember to familiarise yourself with and adhere to the local policy of the trust or organisation that you are working for. If you are unsure what you are permitted to do, discuss this immediately with your supervisor or line manager. Similarly, if you are unsure about the ethical implications of something, you should meet with your supervisor or line manager before taking action; this also applies for safeguarding concerns. Doing so will demonstrate that you are a safe practitioner and can identify the boundaries of your scope of practice, as well as the valuable contributions you make to the MDT. In any clinical environment you work in, ensure that your documentation is consistently of the highest standards. Clear and concise documentation enables effective communication and mitigates risk to patients. To reiterate a self-assessment method of your documentation, if you could read your documentation in ten years' time and understand what happened in the events you have written about, your documentation is detailed enough. Always remember to be objective in your documentation, as patients or their family members may see it at some time.

Activities: Brief outline answers

Activity 3.2 Critical thinking (page 47)

The correlations between the Health and Social Care Act fact sheets (GOV.UK, 2012) and the *Standards of Proficiency for Nursing Associates* (NMC, 2018a) are:

- Need for improvement / Platform 5: Improving safety and quality of care
- Greater voice for patients (Part 5) / Platform 3: Provide and monitor care
- Greater accountability locally and nationally (Parts 1 and 5) / Platform 1: Being an accountable professional.

This is not a definitive list, so you may have identified other links between these two documents. Discuss your answers with your supervisor or line manager in clinical practice to explore your thoughts.

Activity 3.3 Evidence-based practice and research (page 47)

According to the NHS (2018b), some examples of situations or conditions where the Mental Capacity (Amendment) Act 2019 is needed to protect people are:

- dementia;
- severe learning disability;
- brain injury;
- mental health condition;
- stroke.

Activity 3.7 Critical thinking and reflection (page 52)

This activity is challenging, and the situation is common in clinical practice. Evidently, Thomas' children care about their father and are likely to feel upset if he decides to sign a DNAR form. In the activity, it is explained that Thomas has mental capacity, so he is legally able to make this decision independently. He may decide to discuss this with his family, but they cannot force him to sign or not sign a DNAR form. With regard to an ethical theory or framework, one of Beauchamp and Childress' (2013) principles of biomedical ethics is to have respect for autonomy. This principle is directly relevant to Thomas' situation because he has mental capacity. While your role as a nursing associate is to care for the patient, empowering them to make a decision independently, your duty of care also includes the patient's family, friends and carers. It is important to recognise the therapeutic and emotional support that Thomas' family may need. You may be asked to accompany your supervisor to advise the family what support is available to them (e.g. counselling). By providing this support, you are ensuring that you are providing person-centred care to both Thomas and his family, despite them all having different care needs. Always remember to ask your supervisor or another experienced colleague to accompany you when speaking with patients and their family, friends and carers about emotive topics, such as end of life, as well as documenting everything clearly in the patient's notes afterwards to ensure accurate record-keeping.

Activity 3.8 Critical thinking (page 53)

1. *Gillick v West Norfolk and Wisbech Area Health Authority* is a case law that defines what is now known as Gillick competence.

2. Deontology could be applied to this activity because the GP's actions could be seen as being in the best interests for Victoria at that time, despite her mother's disagreement. However, it is important to note that ethical philosophies and frameworks only guide practice, whereas legislation defines what is legal and what is illegal.

3. A potential safeguarding concern depends on the context of the situation. If Victoria booked an appointment to see her GP without her parents to discuss contraception because she was embarrassed and there were no issues at home, there is no safeguarding concern. However, if Victoria booked the appointment with her GP without her parents and said this was because she was unsafe and/or being abused at home, there would be a safeguarding concern. Safeguarding requires careful thought due to the potential complexity of this situation, so if you have a safeguarding concern ensure that you speak with your supervisor or line manager immediately. Make sure that you are fully aware of your local trust's policy on safeguarding, as this will inform your practice in these circumstances.

Annotated further reading

Beauchamp, T. and Childress, J. (2013) *Principles of Biomedical Ethics*, 7th edition. Oxford: Oxford University Press.

This is a seminal textbook on biomedical ethics. As you can see, this book has been republished several times, which is evidence of the validity and reliability of the content. You should be able to access a copy via your local or hospital library.

GOV.UK (2012) *Health and Social Care Act 2012 Fact Sheets*. Available at: www.gov.uk/government/publications/health-and-social-care-act-2012-fact-sheets

This is a list of short fact sheets that are freely available for you to read. They contain specific information about the Health and Social Care Act 2012, so you can download only the information you need.

GOV.UK (2020) *Department of Health and Social Care*. Available at: www.gov.uk/government/organisations/department-of-health-and-social-care

Visit this web page to set up an email alert regarding laws and other news from the Department of Health and Social Care. This will help you to stay up to date with changes in the law.

Griffith, R. and Tengnah, C. (2020) *Law and Professional Issues in Nursing*, 5th edition. London: SAGE.

This book provides you with an overview of all law that is relevant to the nursing professions, which will inform your practice as a nursing associate. The authors have purposefully written it in accessible language and the book content is comprehensive. The case studies included in the book support you to understand how law is applied to different situations in clinical practice.

King's Fund (2016) *House of Commons Health Committee Inquiry on Public Health Post-2013: Evidence Submission*. Available at: www.kingsfund.org.uk/publications/submission-health-committee-inquiry-public-health

This web page takes you to the submission of evidence about the impact of the Health and Social Care Act 2012. There is a summary and an extended version for you to read.

UK Parliament (2019) *How Are Laws Made?* Available at: www.parliament.uk/about/how/laws/

For a short video explanation on the process of how laws are created, watch the video that can be found on this web page.

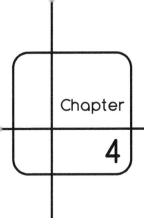

Palliative and end of life care

Chapter aims

After reading this chapter, you will be able to:

- assess the needs of a dying patient;
- recognise when and how to adjust communication techniques and person-centred care for a dying patient;

(Continued)

(Continued)

- know how to support a dying patient's family, friends and carers, as well as involving them in the patient's care, where appropriate;
- understand the relevant legislation for patients who are dying.

Introduction

As you are aware, nursing associates are generalist practitioners and are unique professionals within the MDT. The unique factors are that your pre-registration education includes all four fields of nursing and caring for patients across their lifespan. Evidently, the care of a patient who is at the end of their life is an integral part of your clinical practice. **End of life** care is defined as care that takes place during the last year of a patient's life. It is always a doctor (or an appropriately qualified practitioner) who formally identifies that a patient has entered end of life care, but, where possible and appropriate, family, friends and carers are also involved in this process. In reality, diagnosing that a patient has entered end of life care can be challenging or unpredictable. Throughout this chapter, you will be able to define dying and have an awareness of what stage of the dying process a patient is in. It is important to remember that patients can die at any stage of their lifespan, depending on the condition(s) they have. This chapter will guide you in recognising your role as a nursing associate during end of life care, as well as how you can provide person-centred care for the dying. It is always important to involve the patient's family, friends and carers (i.e. anyone who is important to them) in their care. Death will change their relationship, and they will have needs too, so you have a duty of care to them as well as to the patient. This chapter will help you to do this. Lastly, this chapter will link with Chapter 3, highlighting specific legislation that you need to be aware of which relates to end of life care and death. Although thinking about death may seem like a depressing or morbid subject, end of life care is an opportunity to provide the last best quality person-centred care a patient will have before they die. This is a huge privilege and will make a lifelong impact on the patient's family and friends if their experience of end of life care is positive.

Defining death and dying

The terms 'palliative care' and 'end of life care' are commonly used interchangeably; however, there is a difference between the two. Palliative care is in fact the treatment of a patient with a life-limiting illness (Marie Curie, 2018a). Usually, life-limiting illnesses are long-term conditions that prevent a patient from carrying out their typical daily routine. Of course, everyone's daily routines are different; therefore, healthcare professionals can use a theory called the Roper-Logan-Tierney model of nursing, also known as the activities of daily living (ADLs) (Roper et al., 2000). Roper et al. (2000) state that there are 12 ADLs which people experience across their lifespan:

- maintaining a safe environment;
- communication;
- breathing;
- eating and drinking;
- elimination;
- washing and dressing;
- controlling temperature;

- mobilisation;
- working and playing;
- expressing sexuality;
- sleeping;
- death and dying.

When a patient is receiving palliative care, it does not mean that they cannot do one (or more) of the 12 ADLs, but their abilities are limited due to their long-term condition. Furthermore, some of the ADLs are not completely relevant to palliative care. Sudden death, for example, is not within the speciality of palliative care, whereas someone who has limited breathing due to having chronic obstructive pulmonary disease (COPD) would constitute palliative care. Other conditions that require the patient to have palliative care would be dementia, cancer or Huntington's disease (Marie Curie, 2018a).

Palliative care is not limited to the patient. Their family, friends and carers are also included in palliative care, so it is truly holistic. Practitioners who specialise in this area aim to improve the quality of a patient's life as much as possible while managing their life-limiting illness. This can include physiological symptoms, psychosocial and spiritual needs, and social care for the patient, as well as for the family or friends who look after them. Other members of the MDT may need to complete specialist assessments to meet these needs. For example, occupational therapists can assess how safe the patient's home is for them to live in, which links with the ADLs mentioned earlier. Also mentioned earlier is the use of palliative care to replace end of life care. Strictly speaking, they can be the same thing. If a patient has begun to die, and it is not a rapid death, the patient will experience a limitation in their typical ADLs. In context, think about a patient who has end-stage pancreatic cancer. They may have one or two months left to live. During this time, their ability to carry out ADLs will deteriorate, and it is the palliative care specialist's responsibility to meet the patient's needs, including the needs of their family, friends and carers. At this point, the patient with pancreatic cancer is receiving both palliative care and end of life care. With this in mind, what is the definition of end of life care?

End of life care occurs during the last 12 months of a patient's life and is therefore an integral part of palliative care (Marie Curie, 2018a). Determining when a patient enters the last year of their life can be difficult. Every patient has a different dying process (e.g. patients die at different speeds depending on their health and life-limiting illnesses). The aim of end of life care is to ensure that the patient is as comfortable as possible. By definition, end of life care also includes family, friends and carers because these people are important to the patient. Similar to palliative care, end of life care is holistic and includes physical and psychological health. For some patients and their family and friends, religious needs may also be very significant. You can read more about meeting religious needs later in this chapter. If you would like to read more about the difference between palliative care and end of life care, the charity Marie Curie is a fantastic, freely available resource. You can find links to the Marie Curie website in the annotated further reading section at the end of the chapter, which you will need to complete Activity 4.1.

Activity 4.1　Research

There are many misconceptions about palliative care and end of life care. It is important for you as a nursing associate to have a clear understanding of the differences, as well as being able to answer any questions that a patient or their family, friends and carers may have. The Marie Curie website is full of very useful information about palliative care and end of life care.

(Continued)

(Continued)

Researching this information and keeping yourself up to date is important for you to be able to provide person-centred care. For this activity, visit the first Marie Curie web page in the annotated further reading section at the end of the chapter and search for 'common myths about palliative care' (Marie Curie, 2018a, p1). Make a note of these myths and try to remember them, as these are questions that patients or their family and friends may ask you.

Not only could you do your own research using the Marie Curie website, but you could signpost it to patients and their family, friends and carers as a reliable source of information. It is important to highlight reliable sources to patients, particularly if they have just received some unexpected news.

An outline answer is provided at the end of the chapter.

Completing Activity 4.1 will provide you with reliable information that you can share with patients and their family, friends and carers when they ask questions about their palliative care. The answers about myths and facts provided at the end of the chapter are cited from the Marie Curie website, but remember that information is regularly updated, so do not rely on the answers provided here. Go to the website to check if it has been updated so that you are fully up to date about the differences between palliative care and end of life care.

This chapter focuses on end of life care, which we now know is an integral part of palliative care. This may lead you to question, 'How do doctors know if a patient has begun the last year of their life, and what are the stages of dying?' The Marie Curie website has information for patients and their family and friends, as mentioned before; however, it also has sections for healthcare professionals. The second Marie Curie web page in the annotated further reading section at the end of the chapter will bring you to the healthcare professionals page (Marie Curie, 2018b, p1). To summarise this information, there are a number of physiological and psychological changes that a patient experiences as they begin the last days and hours of their life. Some examples might be that their ADLs become progressively more limited, they may tell you that they feel like they are dying, and towards the last few hours their breathing pattern may change and become more laboured. You may also hear a snoring-like sound during the last few hours of a patient's life, which is called **agonal breathing**. This is not the same as snoring, and it has a unique sound.

It is important to note that patients may have varied signs and symptoms when they are in the last days or hours of their life. Furthermore, the dying process may be quicker for some patients and slower for others. Communication between the patient, and their family, friends, carers and healthcare professionals is paramount. It is of the upmost importance that a palliative care specialist practitioner has a discussion with the patient and their loved ones about what their preferences are. Some preferences may be based on religious, cultural or spiritual beliefs, which will be discussed later in this chapter. The patient's wishes should be clearly documented and shared with the MDT so that person-centred care can be provided. With this in mind, what is your role as a nursing associate?

The nursing associate's role in person-centred end of life care

If a patient is known to be unwell and is expected to need end of life care in the near future, monitor any changes in their ADLs. An example from practice may be a patient who has been diagnosed with stage 4 (end-stage) cancer. If you notice changes in their ADLs, do not discuss this with the patient or their family and friends at this stage. The initial conversation about end of life care must be completed by a palliative care specialist. However, if you do notice changes, report this to the patient's GP, their district nurse team or, most importantly, their palliative care team (Marie Curie, 2018b). The palliative care team will be able to meet the specific needs of the patient as they begin their last days of life. It is imperative that this referral is made as early as possible so that there is adequate time to complete a holistic assessment and meet the needs of the patient and their family, friends and carers. Sometimes the signs and symptoms that appear to be end of life can be as a result of other conditions that are manageable. For example, a chest infection will change a patient's respiratory pattern whether they are palliative or simply have an alternative acute or long-term condition. Medical staff in the palliative care team will make this diagnosis, but remember that you, as a nursing associate, spend a lot of time with patients, so it is likely that you will notice changes in their ADLs first.

The *Standards of Proficiency for Nursing Associates* state that you need to be able to demonstrate and understand how to provide holistic care to a patient during end of life care (NMC, 2018a). As previously mentioned, the diagnosis and initial conversation about end of life care will be completed by the palliative care team in the service that you work in. They will put together a care plan, similarly to a patient with an acute or long-term condition. Your role as a nursing associate providing end of life care therefore mirrors your person-centred approach to caring for a patient with an acute or long-term condition. Remember that the nursing process is a generic framework which can be applied in any care environment (Howatson-Jones et al., 2015). However, as well as providing physical care to patients, the other components of holistic care are extremely significant, particularly educating patients about their condition and what to expect next (if they want to know). Chapter 7 is partly about patient education, but in the meantime complete Activity 4.2 as it will provide you with some guidance on how to maintain effective communication.

Activity 4.2   Research

Via the same web page mentioned in Activity 4.1, there is a video that focuses on what to expect at the end of life (Marie Curie, 2018a). A Marie Curie nurse discusses the importance of understanding the process and stages of dying during the last weeks, days and hours of a patient's life. This video provides patients with an additional source of information about their care; however, it can also be watched by you, as a nursing associate, to inform your knowledge of end of life care.

When a patient is diagnosed with a terminal illness, it is evidently a shock. Although the patient's consultant or palliative care team may explain everything in detail, the patient and their family and friends may not be able to remember what was said due to the shock. Another role of the nursing associate, therefore, could be to reiterate what the consultant or palliative care team have said. When doing this, you could signpost the video found via the web page mentioned at the beginning of this activity. Although it may seem like the same information is being repeated, a consistent message will be reassuring for the patient and their family, friends and carers. Furthermore, knowing that there is a valid and reliable information and advice service, such as Marie Curie, available to them will reduce the stress of trying to remember large volumes of information. Watch this video before going into practice so that you are fully informed of the information available to patients. Always remember that websites are regularly updated, so you need to ensure that your knowledge and clinical practice are based on current evidence.

As this activity is based on your own reflection, there is no outline answer provided at the end of the chapter.

Activity 4.2 will help you to understand the end of life care process. To ensure that you are providing person-centred end of life care, always complete a holistic assessment and provide care that is bespoke to the needs of the patient you are looking after, including their family, friends and carers. So far in this chapter, it has been discussed that patients will have different signs and symptoms during end of life care, which will occur at different speeds. Another significant difference that is directly relevant to your practice as a nursing associate is the variations of end of life care across the lifespan.

When discussing death, it is usually in reference to adults; however, it is important to know the differences between end of life care for an adult and end of life care for a child or infant. Cancer can affect a person at any stage of their lifespan, and in 2017 it was the leading cause of death for children aged 1–15 years (ONS, 2018). Changes in ADLs take place across a patient's lifespan, and these changes are unique to the patient. However, the age of a child needs to be taken into account to determine the amount of independence considered typical. An infant (aged 0–12 months), for example, is completely dependent on their parent or guardian, but this is perfectly normal. Changes in what are considered normal ADLs are what should be monitored. The National Institute for Health and Care Excellence (NICE) provides evidence-based guidance for a variety of topics, including end of life care. NICE Pathways provides an interactive web page that provides succinct information about end of life care for people across the lifespan (NICE Pathways, 2019). This is a valid and reliable source of information to inform your practice, so it is worthwhile visiting the website.

Once a patient has died, end of life care does not stop at this point. It is within your scope of practice to care for the deceased's body (NMC, 2018a). Historically, this process was called 'last offices' (which has connotations with Christianity), but guidance published by Hospice UK advocates using the term **'care after death'** because this is more inclusive and representative of our multicultural society (Wilson, 2015). In this guidance, 'care after death' refers to the whole process of caring for the patient's body, as well as their family, friends and carers, whereas the term **'personal care after death'** is used in reference to the physical preparation of the patient's body before being moved to the mortuary or funeral director (Wilson, 2015). The process described in the guidance refers to care after death of an adult. Regardless of how old the deceased was, you should always adhere to your local trust's policy of care after death. However, the process described in the guidance is a useful tool to help you recognise the predominant stages in the process:

1. Death is verified by a qualified practitioner.
2. Personal care after death is when the patient's body is washed and prepared for viewing by the patient's family, friends and carers. Some families may wish to be involved in this part of the process.
3. A medical certificate of cause of death is issued.
4. The patient's body is transferred to the mortuary.
5. The deceased is transported to the funeral director by undertakers.
6. The death is registered and a death certificate is issued by the registrar.
7. The burial or cremation takes place, or the patient's body is donated to medical science, or the patient's body is repatriated abroad to another country – whatever the patient's choice was.

This list includes the predominant steps for care after death; however, there may be some differences in the policies where you work, or the inclusion of special religious, spiritual or cultural needs. For example, in Western culture, many people open a window shortly after the patient has died to allow their spirit to leave. In Judaism, some people place a feather on the patient's lips to further verify their death – if the patient breathes again, the feather will move. In Catholicism, the patient may ask to see a priest in the last few hours of their life. In Islam, the washing of the patient's body after they have died is religiously significant and is completed by the patient's family and friends, as well as an imam. Each religion has different denominations, so religious practices may vary slightly. In addition, when you think about how many religions there are, it is evident why not all religious, spiritual and cultural practices can be mentioned here, although these examples may provide you with some guidance.

It is important to note, however, that although the patient and their family or friends may identify as believing in a particular religion, spirituality or cultural norm, they may practise their beliefs in a different way. Therefore, to ensure that you are providing person-centred care after death, have a discussion with the patient and their family or friends about their preferences. Always make sure you have a registered nurse with you, as you can support each other and demonstrate to the patient and their family and friends that you are working as a team to meet their needs. Another example of when you will need at least two members of staff present is if the patient who is dying (or has died, in some circumstances) is eligible for organ donation.

Organ donation

Organ donation can be defined as when a patient volunteers to donate their organs when they die to another patient who needs an organ replacement. There are many organs that can be donated (e.g. heart, lungs, liver, kidneys, pancreas, small bowel), and some tissues can also be donated (e.g. cornea and bones) (NHS Blood and Transplant, 2020). A patient for whom you are providing end of life care may be eligible to donate their organs when they die; however, there are very clear eligibility criteria that you can read on the NHS Blood and Transplant website (see the annotated further reading section at the end of the chapter). You will not need to discuss organ donation with the patient or their family, friends and carers, because this is always done by an organ donation specialist (usually a nurse). On the other hand, you may be caring for a patient who is waiting for a donated organ. Similarly, you can signpost the NHS Blood and Transplant website as a valid and reliable source of information if a patient or their family, friends and carers would like more information.

In the spring of 2020, a new law introduced in England means that all adults are automatically on the organ donation register. The updated organ donation system in England, also known as Max and Keira's law, means that all adults (aged 18 years or older) need to opt out of the organ donation register if they would prefer that their organs not be donated. This initiative has been introduced to save more lives of patients in desperate need of donated organs. The story behind Max and Keira's law is a clear example of how beneficial organ donation can be; the following case study provides you with more information about Max and Keira.

Case study: Max and Keira

Max is a boy who was diagnosed with cardiomyopathy, a long-term condition affecting his heart muscle. He needed a heart transplant and was added to the organ donation waiting list. During this time, he met other children who had been on the waiting list for much longer and he wanted to help. Max began a campaign in support of the opt-out organ donation system so that it would be easier for people to donate their organs, which would save many lives of people waiting for an eligible organ to be donated. Max was fortunate enough to receive a donated heart from a girl named Keira, who sadly died in a road traffic collision. During recovery, Max continued to share his story to raise awareness of organ donation. In 2018, the government produced a Bill that would change the organ donation process to an opt-out system. Originally, once enacted, the legislation would have been called Max's law; however, Max wanted to include Keira's name, and hence the legislation enacted in spring 2020 was called Max and Keira's law. On the NHS Blood

(Continued)

(Continued)

and Transplant website, you can watch a video of Keira's parents listening to her heart beating inside Max: **www.organdonation.nhs.uk/helping-you-to-decide/real-life-stories/people-who-have-benefitted-from-receiving-a-transplant/max-heart-transplant-recipient-and-campaigner/**

Max and Keira's story is just one example of many patients' stories where organ donation has provided them with a second chance in life. Organ donation is, of course, an emotive subject to discuss, hence why an organ donation specialist always leads this conversation. Some people do not want to donate their organs because of religious, spiritual or cultural beliefs, and this is a decision that we must respect as healthcare professionals. Some patients may want to be organ donors but may have questions about how their religious, spiritual or cultural beliefs will be respected. According to NHS Blood and Transplant (2020), all major religions endorse organ donation in principle; however, organ donation is fundamentally an individual choice. Activity 4.3 helps you to explore more about organ donation and religious beliefs.

Activity 4.3   Research

All religions in the UK support organ donation in principle; however, it is important to note that a patient must make an informed decision about remaining on the organ donation register. The patient may wish to discuss this with their family and friends so that they are aware of their decision, including how their religious beliefs will be respected. The organ donation specialists will have a discussion with the family and friends after the patient dies to ensure that all of their wishes are respected. NHS Blood and Transplant (2020) provides answers to questions about organ donation and religion, faith and beliefs. Use this information to answer the following questions:

1. How can patients ensure that their religion, faith and beliefs are respected if they choose to remain on the organ donation register?
2. How can patients request an organ donation specialist with whom to discuss their wishes, as well as those of their family and friends?
3. If the patient changes their mind about organ donation, how can this be recognised?
4. What should a patient do if they decide to remain opted in on the organ donation register but their family disagrees that their religion, faith or beliefs endorse organ donation?

An outline answer is provided at the end of the chapter.

As discussed in this section, Max and Keira's law will legally change the organ donation process to an opt-out system. There are other laws related to palliative and end of life care that you should also have an awareness of.

Laws related to palliative and end of life care

There are many laws that are related to palliative and end of life care – more than can be discussed in this chapter. However, some legislation has been included to highlight examples of laws you need to have awareness of.

Part of palliative and end of life care focuses on planning for the future. An early holistic assessment is critical to ensure that patients' decisions are respected, and thus person-centred care can be achieved. A key example of when this is necessary could be when a patient is diagnosed with a type of **dementia**. Some literature suggests that there are as many as 400 different types of dementia, but common types are Alzheimer's disease, vascular dementia and Lewy body dementia (Dementia: Understand Together, 2020). Another type is called early onset dementia, which, as the name suggests, can be diagnosed in people from the age of 40 years old. For patients with early onset dementia, their functionality progressively deteriorates and eventually they will be unsafe to make decision for themselves. Before this eventuality, there should be a legal process to identify a member of the patient's family as a lasting power of attorney (although this can be a patient's friend, if they prefer).

Someone that is a lasting power of attorney has the legal right to make decisions on behalf of the patient regarding their personal welfare and/or their property and financial affairs (Age UK, 2019a). There are lasting power of attorney subcategories, which you can find out more about via the Age UK web page in the annotated further reading section at the end of the chapter. This legal empowerment is enforced via the Mental Capacity (Amendment) Act 2019, discussed in Chapter 3. In the context of palliative and end of life care for someone that has early onset dementia, once they no longer have mental capacity their lasting power of attorney can then step in to make decisions on their behalf. This does not mean that the patient's opinion is ignored; their previous and current wishes are included as much as possible, where it is safe to do so. Before reading more about the law that applies to palliative and end of life care, complete Activity 4.4 to learn more about a patient's perspective of living with dementia.

Activity 4.4   Reflection

In 2007, a book called *Still Alice* was published, written by Lisa Genova, a story about the life of Professor Alice Howland at Harvard University who is diagnosed with early onset dementia in her early fifties. Although this book is a novel, not an academic text, the narrative provides a very sincere account of what it is like to live with a degenerative disease such as dementia. As healthcare professionals, we can become immune to the impact that acute and long-term conditions actually have on patients, particularly if we have never been patients ourselves. Reading *Still Alice* is one way to understand patients' perspectives and have empathy for their condition, as well as their families, friends and carers. If your learning preference is more visual, *Still Alice* was adapted into a film in 2014.

After reading the book or seeing the film, reflect on what you have learned from this story and how you may change your practice as a result. Discuss this learning with your supervisor or line manager, and if they are unaware of the story recommend that they read the book and/or watch the film.

As this activity is based on your own reflection, there is no outline answer provided at the end of the chapter.

Although Activity 4.4 is based on a novel, there is valuable learning from the characters' narratives, particularly from the protagonist, Professor Alice Howland. Her story may raise questions about what her thoughts were during her palliative and end of life care. One question might be whether she considered seeking euthanasia or assisted suicide. Many patients or their family, friends and carers may discuss this, as well as having signs and symptoms of depression. It is important for you as a nursing associate to know about relevant legislation in this area.

Euthanasia can be defined as deliberately ending a patient's life who has a terminal illness and is treated as manslaughter or murder – the maximum sentence is 14 years' imprisonment. Assisted suicide, on the other hand, can be defined as the deliberate act of someone enabling or encouraging a patient with a terminal illness to commit suicide. Assisted suicide is also illegal, as enforced by the Suicide Act 1961. These laws are very clear in their content; however, many people debate whether assisted suicide should be legalised. A small number of other countries around the world do permit assisted suicide, but this practice is only legalised if very strict eligibility criteria are met. Many people have strong views on assisted suicide founded on religious, spiritual or cultural beliefs. You may also have strong opinions on this topic. Of course, it is important that when working as a nursing associate, your thoughts, biases or subjectivity do not have an effect on the care you are providing. As previously mentioned in Chapter 1, person-centred care, include palliative and end of life care, must be legal, equal and in accordance with *The Code* (NMC, 2018b).

The laws discussed in this section are not a complete list of the legislation you need to have an awareness of. With this in mind, you may want to include researching palliative and end of life care laws to your CPD goals or your annual appraisal.

Supporting the patient's family, friends and carers after the patient has died

During this chapter, there have been many examples and references to explain how to involve the patient's family, friends and carers in end of life care. Once the patient has died, care of the patient's loved ones continues, and thus you will be ensuring continuity of care after death. It is obvious to say that the patient's family, friends and carers will need emotional support during end of life care, as well as after the patient has died, but what other care do they need?

Even if a patient's death is expected, the shock when it does happen can cause their family, friends and carers to feel a sense of loss and confusion. Even if they have discussed what they need to do, the emotions felt can be overwhelming. Once a patient has died, it is important to offer their family, friends and carers time alone with the patient. Other family members or friends may visit the patient, which is an important first step in the grieving process. After you have provided care after death, with or without the patient's family and friends, they may ask you what the next steps are. It is highly important to communicate effectively and, if necessary, explain the next steps in different ways.

You may need to explain that once care after death has been provided, the patient's body will be transported to the mortuary or funeral director, where the patient's body will similarly be cared for. Reiterating the continuity of care after death may help the patient's family, friends and carers to feel reassured, which will allow them to begin the grieving process. You may then need to explain (or re-explain) steps 3–7 from the Hospice UK guidance discussed earlier in this chapter (Wilson, 2015). Remember that you can signpost valid and reliable resources to the patient's family and friends so that they can go back to this information later. It is sensible to write this down for them to reduce the risk of them forgetting what you have said. The service you work for may have information leaflets, so make sure to also offer these to the patient's family, friends and carers. Many health and social care services offer counselling to those who have experienced the death of a loved one, also known as grief counselling. Only signpost information that you know is valid and reliable. In other words, check to see if where you work has a grief counselling service before offering this.

Supporting colleagues' and your own needs when providing end of life care

Caring for patients at the end of their lives is upsetting for their family, friends and carers, but you need to remember that you and your colleagues may also need to process this experience. Professionalism was discussed in Chapter 1, which involves treating patients equally and as individuals. However, it can be very difficult to suppress our own emotions when caring for people during end of life. A patient may remind you of one of your own family or friends who has died, which will inevitably surface your own grief, and similarly a colleague may experience similar emotions to you. To uphold the principles of professionalism in *The Code*, it is important to take time out to discuss and reflect on care that affects you personally (NMC, 2018b).

Professionalism during end of life care is a grey area. For example, crying hysterically when the patient dies in front of their family and friends would be unprofessional; however, allowing yourself to have empathy with their family, friends and carers is professional. No one is expected to suppress their emotions, so if you do feel you need to take a step back, discuss this with a colleague at the earliest possible moment so that they can step in. Take yourself away from the patient's environment and find your manager or a senior colleague to discuss your thoughts. This is perfectly natural, and by doing so you will be demonstrating true professionalism. Once you have gathered your thoughts, you can return to the clinical environment. Additionally, having protected time for a reflective discussion will also enable the team to process a highly emotive part of their job. This does not need to be an extensively long conversation, but it should be led by a senior or experienced member of the team. Identifying the strengths and areas for improvement regarding person-centred end of life care will help everyone to reflect and process their thoughts.

Chapter summary

This chapter is very important for you as a nursing associate. There is only one opportunity to care well for someone at the end of their life. As nursing associates provide care across patients' lifespans, you can make extremely meaningful contributions to the provision of person-centred end of life care, informed by the MDT holistic assessment. End of life care also involves the patient's family, friends and carers, and it is important to involve them wherever appropriate. Your advanced communication skills will be needed here to ensure that person-centred care is provided and no miscommunication occurs. Remember the difference between end of life and palliative care, as this will determine the care interventions you provide. Lastly, remember to look after yourself. Providing end of life care can be very emotionally stressful, particularly if you are in a long-term care setting and have a rapport with a patient who is dying. Always be professional with patients and their family, friends and carers, but allow yourself some time to reflect and discuss your thoughts and feelings with a trusted colleague and/or your supervisor or line manager. Recognising that you have done everything possible to ensure that the patient received person-centred care will be a comforting thought. For more details on looking after yourself, see Chapter 8.

Activities: Brief outline answers

Activity 4.1 Research (page 59)

- *Myth*: 'If I need palliative care, it means that I'll have to go to a hospice.'
- *Fact*: You can receive palliative care in a range of settings, including your home, a hospital, a care home or a hospice.
- *Myth*: 'If I have palliative care, it means that my doctors have given up and I'll no longer receive active treatment for my illness.'
- *Fact*: You can receive palliative care alongside treatments for your illness, such as chemotherapy and radiotherapy.
- *Myth*: 'Having palliative care means that I'm going to die soon.'
- *Fact*: You can receive palliative care at any point in your illness. Some people receive palliative care for years, while others will receive care in their last weeks or days.
- *Myth*: 'If I have palliative care, I'll no longer be seen by other specialists who know about my particular disease.'
- *Fact*: You can receive palliative care alongside care from the specialists who have been treating your particular illness.
- *Myth*: 'Palliative care is just about treating pain and other physical symptoms.'
- *Fact*: Palliative care aims to provide a holistic approach to give you the best quality of life possible. This means caring for all your physical, emotional, psychological, social and other needs.
- *Myth*: 'Palliative care isn't for family and friends.'
- *Fact*: Palliative care teams are aware that your illness may have a big impact on your family members and friends. Palliative care teams do what they can to help people cope.

Activity 4.3 Research (page 64)

1. During the registration process, there is a specific question that provides space for the patient to express specific faith or religious beliefs that they would like to be respected should their organs be needed for donation: **www.organdonation.nhs.uk/register-your-decision/register-your-details/**

2. As part of the registration process, the patient may request that an organ donation specialist discusses their wishes with their family and perhaps their religious or faith leader. The organ donation specialist will meet with the patient's family and friends regardless, but answering this question in the online registration provides a platform to make specific requests.

3. If the patient changes their mind about organ donation, even if it is a small change, they can amend their decisions via an online form on the NHS Blood and Transplant website: **www.organdonation.nhs.uk/register-your-decision/amend-your-details/**

4. As in all palliative and end of life care, families, friends and carers are involved as much as possible, providing that the patient provides informed consent for this (see Chapter 3). If they feel that the patient's faith or religion does not endorse organ donation, a meeting with a religious or faith leader can be arranged to discuss these concerns.

Annotated further reading

Age UK (2019) *Power of Attorney*. Available at: www.ageuk.org.uk/information-advice/money-legal/legal-issues/power-of-attorney/

Visit this web page for more information on what a patient's lasting power of attorney is allowed to do. The Age UK website also contains other useful information for clinical practitioners and patients. For example, patients or their family, friends and carers may benefit from Age UK's charitable services or the resources on their website.

Grant, A. and Goodman, B. (2019) *Communication and Interpersonal Skills in Nursing*, 4th edition. London: SAGE.

Interpersonal skills and communication techniques are vital in the provision of person-centred care. However, in palliative and end of life care, these skills are imperative, so this book is an essential addition to your reading list. It is pragmatically structured and discusses many perspectives of interpersonal skills and communication techniques. Now in its fourth edition, it has withstood the test of time and can be seen as a reliable resource.

Marie Curie (2018) *What Are Palliative Care and End of Life Care?* Available at: www.mariecurie.org.uk/help/support/diagnosed/recent-diagnosis/palliative-care-end-of-life-care

This web page defines the differences between palliative and end of life care. This is a useful source of information for you to keep your knowledge up to date, and includes the video mentioned in Activity 4.2. The Marie Curie website is an excellent source of information to signpost to patients. Remember to emphasise to patients, as well as their family and friends, that this website is a valid and reliable source of information for them.

Marie Curie (2018) *Signs That Someone Is in Their Last Days or Hours of Life*. Available at: www.mariecurie.org.uk/professionals/palliative-care-knowledge-zone/final-days/recognising-deterioration-dying-phase

The Marie Curie website has a whole section designated to healthcare professionals that provides in-depth information about palliative care and end of life care, as well as the services that Marie Curie offers and an option to sign up to email notifications.

NHS Blood and Transplant (2020) *Get the Facts About Organ Donation*. Available at: www.organdonation.nhs.uk/helping-you-to-decide/about-organ-donation/get-the-facts/

Use this web page to find a succinct fact sheet about organ donation. You can explore the website too, which has self-guided teaching resources that you can use to consolidate your knowledge of organ donation.

NHS England (2020) *Personalised End of Life Care*. Available at: www.england.nhs.uk/eolc/personalised-care/

NHS England has useful information for you and patients regarding personalised end of life care. There are also links to other related topics that will guide you in providing person-centred palliative and end of life care for patients.

Nicol, J. and Nyatanga, B. (2017) *Palliative and End of Life Care in Nursing*, 2nd edition. London: SAGE.

This book examines the essential components of palliative and end of life care from a nursing perspective. Although mapped for pre-registration nursing students, nursing associates are a nursing profession that can make valuable contributions to providing person-centred palliative and end of life care.

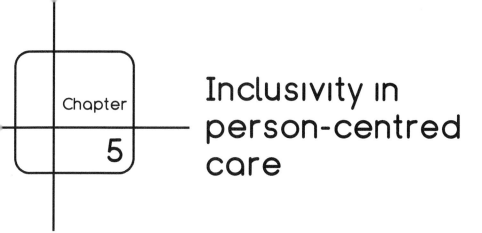

Chapter 5

Inclusivity in person-centred care

NMC *STANDARDS OF PROFICIENCY FOR NURSING ASSOCIATES*

This chapter will address the following platforms and proficiencies:

Platform 1: Being an accountable professional

At the point of registration, the nursing associate will be able to:

1.15 take responsibility for continuous self-reflection, seeking and responding to support and feedback to develop professional knowledge and skills

Platform 3: Provide and monitor care

At the point of registration, the nursing associate will be able to:

3.4   demonstrate the knowledge, communication and relationship management skills required to provide people, families and carers with accurate information that meets their needs before, during and after a range of interventions

3.8   demonstrate and apply an understanding of how people's needs for safety, dignity, privacy, comfort and sleep can be met

3.20 understand and apply the principles and processes for making reasonable adjustments

3.22 recognise when capacity has changed and understand where and how to seek guidance and support from others to ensure that the best interests of those receiving care are upheld

Platform 4: Working in teams

At the point of registration, the nursing associate will be able to:

4.7   support, supervise and act as a role model to nursing associate students, health care support workers and those new to care roles, review the quality of the care they provide, promoting reflection and providing constructive feedback

4.8   contribute to team reflection activities, to promote improvements in practice and services

Chapter aims

After reading this chapter, you will be able to:

- recognise individuality and protected characteristics of patients and their family and friends;
- identify what constitutes a reasonable adjustment to accommodate individual needs;
- consolidate your reflective practice and encourage others to do the same;
- recognise when to ask for advice or guidance from senior and experienced practitioners.

Introduction

Providing person-centred care can only be achieved by practising with inclusivity. The nine protected characteristics of the Equality Act 2010 previously cited in Chapter 3 will be the framework for this chapter. Being able to recognise patients' individuality and their specific needs, as well as including the needs of their family, friends and carers, is paramount to be able to achieve person-centred care. The Equality Act 2010 is a useful guide for you in clinical practice to be able to do this. However, you will also be able to think critically about how reasonable adjustments can be made, as well as identifying when all reasonable adjustments have been attempted. Consolidating your reflective practice is integral to this chapter. Furthermore, the importance of encouraging other healthcare practitioners to adopt reflective practice is also included. Linking with Chapter 3, the principles of mental capacity and informed consent will also be developed in this chapter. In summary, this chapter aims to support you in consolidating the knowledge and skills that you have developed so far, as well as applying them in different contexts and situations. For a refresher on the Equality Act 2010, see the following box.

Understanding the theory: Equality Act 2010

The Equality Act 2010 was originally discussed in Chapter 3. This box can be used to refresh your knowledge of the Equality Act 2010, as well as providing a little more context, as the nine protected characteristics are used as a framework for this chapter.

According to the Equality and Human Rights Commission (2019a), the Equality Act 2010 brought 116 pieces of legislation into one Act of Parliament (you can also see a list of the nine previous legislations via Equality and Human Rights Commission, 2019a). The aim of the Equality Act 2010 is to provide legal protection and equal opportunity for everyone in the UK, regardless of their heritage, background or beliefs. It prevents people from discriminating against someone that has one or more of the nine protected characteristics: age, disability, gender reassignment, marriage or civil partnership, pregnancy and maternity, race, religion or belief, sex, and sexual orientation.

Although the majority of people do not discriminate against anyone intentionally, more knowledge about protected characteristics will increase your awareness of patients with specific needs. A heightened knowledge will enable you to make reasonable adjustments to meet the needs of patients with a protected characteristic, thus naturally providing person-centred care. As a result, patients and their family and friends will feel at ease in your care, and, as discussed in Chapter 1, establishing a rapport with patients is integral to providing person-centred care.

Complete Activity 5.1 to test your understanding of the Equality Act 2010.

Activity 5.1   Critical thinking

How does the Equality Act 2010 apply to your role as a nursing associate when providing person-centred care?

An outline answer is provided at the end of the chapter.

You can find out much more about the Equality Act 2010 by reading the guidance written by the Equality and Human Rights Commission (2019b). Before continuing, you need to understand what the Equality Act 2010 protects people with a protected characteristic from.

Discrimination

In the Equality Act 2010, there are four types of discrimination that are defined:

- *Direct discrimination*: Deliberate maltreatment of someone who has a protected characteristic that results in unfair treatment.
- *Indirect discrimination*: An act that unfairly benefits some people but excludes others who have a protected characteristic.
- *Harassment*: The continued act of belittling, humiliating or intimidating someone with a protected characteristic.
- *Victimisation*: Unfair treatment directed at someone who has raised concerns (or intends to) about discrimination against themselves or another person.

You may be familiar with these terms from your mandatory training in the healthcare service that you work for. It is important to be able to recognise the differences between discrimination so that you can escalate any concerns you have to your supervisor or line manager. Remember to have this conversation in a private space, without an audience and away from the patient and their family and friends. This will reduce the risk of breaching confidentiality (NMC, 2018b).

Moving forward, you now have an understanding of the Equality Act 2010 and the definition of discrimination. The next part of this chapter is separated into short sections as per the nine protected characteristics of the Equality Act 2010. Read on to learn more about how each section relates to inclusivity in person-centred care and your practice as a nursing associate.

1. Age

Some people may be discriminated against due to their age, because they are considered too young or old. As part of your role as a nursing associate, you need to proactively prevent age discrimination against patients and their family and friends. This also includes your colleagues – also known as the public sector equality duty (Age UK, 2019b). An example from clinical practice may be a patient in their mid-60s prevented from consenting to having an operation by their family because they believe that the patient is too old. Not only does this breach the principles of informed consent (see Chapter 3), but the patient is being discriminated against due to their age. This situation may not be as simple as it seems, as there may be other influencing factors behind the scenes that you are unaware of. Nevertheless, in a similar situation, you would discuss this with your supervisor or line manager straight away. They will then enable the patient to have protected space and time to make their own decision, possibly in conversation with the surgeon or their consultant. Complete Activity 5.2 to apply these principles to a clinically based scenario.

Activity 5.2   Critical thinking

Nursing associates are generalist practitioners, and this scope of practice is extremely beneficial when working in any environment that provides care for a large variety of people. Imagine that you are working in a bedded ward environment on a surgical unit. A patient named Raheel is due to be admitted to the ward for surgery on his wrist – he broke his scaphoid by tripping on a pavement curb. Raheel has just had his eighteenth birthday. He has severe autism, attends a specialised school, and is well cared for at home by his parents, James and Yasmine. Legally speaking, Raheel is an adult, but due to his additional learning needs he has the mind of a 3-year-old child. Raheel's parents have requested for him to be admitted to the paediatric ward because they have better facilities to meet his autism needs.

Having Raheel's best interests at the forefront of your mind, should he be admitted to the adult or paediatric ward? Discuss your thoughts with your supervisor or line manager and provide some rationale.

An outline answer is provided at the end of the chapter.

Activity 5.2 links with Chapter 4 because Raheel's situation has legal and ethical considerations. You will need to use your critical thinking skills to take into account the legal and ethical perspectives. Rashly making a judgement without investing time to make an evidence-based decision does not put Raheel's best interests at the centre of your thoughts, whereas making an informed, shared decision with Raheel and his family meets the standards of person-centred care. However, age is only one protected characteristic. Read on to learn about the other protected characteristics and how they affect inclusivity in person-centred care.

2. Disability

In the Equality Act 2010, disability is defined as any substantial and long-term condition that has a negative impact on someone's activities of daily living (GOV.UK, 2020a). See the annotated further reading section at the end of the chapter for a web page that explains in more detail the terms 'substantial' and 'long-term' with regard to disability. In short, 'substantial' means having a significant impact and 'long-term' means 12 months or more. (Linking back to Chapter 1, 'chronic' is defined as six months or longer. 'Long-term', in the context of the Equality Act 2010, is defined as 12 months or longer, so remember not to confuse the two terms.)

A disability can be a physical or psychological condition, and in addition they can be stable or progressive (a condition that becomes worse overtime). Some examples are learning disabilities (as referred to in Activity 5.2), **Huntington's disease**, HIV/AIDS and cancer. Whether a patient has a physical or psychological disability, as healthcare practitioners we must ensure that our clinical practice includes meeting their additional needs. Think back to Chapter 3 in reference to mental capacity. If a patient is protected under the Mental Capacity (Amendment) Act 2019, you can still include them in a decision about their care as much as possible, even though their lasting power of attorney is legally responsible for making safe decisions on their behalf. The rationale for this is that patients who are protected under the Mental Capacity (Amendment) Act 2019 may have days where their mental capacity is better, so it should be presumed that patients have mental capacity, and if their capacity shows signs of change then they need to have another assessment. Furthermore, including them in decisions will help to reduce anxiety and frustration, and thus you would be providing inclusive person-centred care.

The next section focuses on three protected characteristics that are closely related to one another, so they have been grouped together for this chapter.

3. Gender reassignment / 4. Sex / 5. Sexual orientation

Before discussing gender reassignment, it is worthwhile defining what the term 'gender' means and how it differs from 'sex', as they are commonly misinterpreted. A person's **sex** is in reference to what physically makes someone male or female (i.e. what genitalia they have). In rare cases, children can be born with both sets of genitalia, although one set is usually more developed than the other. This is known as 'hermaphroditism', although some people prefer the term 'intersex'. However, sex is very different to gender.

Gender refers to the sex that someone identifies as. Statistically, there are more people who identify the same as their sex, but many people feel more comfortable identifying as the opposite of their sex. Some people use the term **'transgender'** to describe their gender identity as the opposite of their sex at birth, but note that being transgender is not a sexuality (see later in this section). In other words, gender is psychological, whereas sex is physiological. It is important to note, however, that gender is not dichotomous (one or the other). A patient you are caring for may feel somewhat like a woman while their sex is male, and vice versa. In reality, this may mean that they feel most comfortable wearing what is typically known as 'female clothing' at work, but when socialising they prefer to wear 'male clothing'. Inverted commas have been used to highlight that clothing is often labelled as male or female; however, this is a social construct (common belief) within cultures and societies. A contextual example from the UK is that traditionally, English, Northern Irish and Welsh men wear trousers or shorts, whereas in formal Scottish attire men sometimes wear kilts, which look similar to skirts, but the social construct in Scotland is that a kilt is a 'masculine' garment, whereas a skirt is often labelled as 'feminine'. So, in other words, clothing does not have a sex; therefore, it is ironic that people label them as 'male' or 'female' in different cultures and societies. The important point to recognise here is how comfortable people feel when identifying as a particular gender, not their choice of clothing. In addition to this, gender identity is not a choice, but an introspective mindset that people discover – or rediscover – over time.

Gender is often described as a choice, but it is more of a fluid spectrum. People take time to realise what makes them feel most comfortable, and this may mean moving along the gender spectrum and back again. In other words, a patient's gender may change over time, and you may notice this if you are working in a long-term care setting. A patient, young or old, may discuss these thoughts and feelings with you if they feel comfortable to do so. However, never initiate this conversation because gender is deeply personal and, as previously mentioned, it takes time to realise what identify feels most comfortable. Another pair of often misused terms that you should have an awareness of are 'sexuality' and 'gender reassignment'.

Sexuality can be defined as the sexual attraction that people feel towards one another. Notice here that sexuality is not related to gender, which, as previously discussed, is to do with sex identity. There are many different types of sexuality (e.g. heterosexual, homosexual), but the health and wellbeing of people is far more of a priority for clinical practitioners in comparison to applying a label. In practice, you may work in a sexual health clinic and provide information about contraception or reducing the risk of sexually transmitted infections/diseases. Similarly, **gender reassignment** is not related to sexuality. Gender reassignment is a process that some people choose to have to change their birth sex; this process can also be called sex reassignment. Gender reassignment involves hormone therapy or surgery, or sometimes both. It is a complex process that takes time. For example, just to be eligible for gender reassignment surgery, a person must live as their preferred gender identity for at least two years (although local policy may differ in some areas, so always check the policy where you are working). In relation to your role as a nursing associate, you may be providing **perioperative** care for patients who are having gender reassignment surgery.

It is important not to confuse the many terms that are commonly misinterpreted. Key terms, as always, are highlighted in bold, and definitions are provided in the glossary at the end of the book. Some examples of your practice as a nursing associate have been mentioned, but these do not include every scenario that you will come across at work. Most people who work in health and social care already have an open mind, but remember to use your active listening skills, apply the principles of person-centred care and take the time to understand each person as an individual. To reiterate a previous learning point, applying a label to someone is not person-centred care, but providing holistic care that meets their needs is. Read the next section to find out about marriage, civil partnership and inclusivity in person-centred care.

6. Marriage and civil partnership

The first question to ask here is: Do you know the difference between marriage and civil partnership? Both are marital statuses and have equal rights in terms of UK law (i.e. people who are in a civil partnership have the same legal protection with regard to their relationship as those who are married) (Citizens Advice, 2020). The legal status of a patient relates to your practice in many ways, but particularly when identifying the patient's next of kin. A patient's next of kin will typically be their husband, wife or civil partner. However, be cautious here not to make presumptions. A patient may decide to have another family member as their next of kin because their husband, wife or civil partner may have additional health needs, such as dementia. As this example demonstrates, be guided by the patient regarding their next of kin; this approach empowers the patient and ensures that they are at the centre of your practice. If you would like to read more about the legal difference between marriage and civil partnership, see the Citizens Advice web page listed in the annotated further reading section at the end of the chapter. This is a useful resource to signpost to patients and their family, friends and carers if they would like more information.

In the UK, it is legal for any man or woman to be married to any other person above the age of legal consent (although people aged 16–17 years require at least one written parental or guardian permission) (Citizens Advice, 2020). Some religious denominations believe that marriage can only be recognised between a man and a woman, and civil partnerships may also not be condoned. This perspective is a philosophical and ethical debate; however, as healthcare practitioners, we must ensure that we respect every person and their beliefs, regardless of whether we share or disagree with them. At this point, think back to the definitions of professionalism in Chapter 1. Your role as a nursing associate is to ensure that all people are respected by yourself and others, which requires you to leave your personal beliefs, perspectives and prejudices at home, as well as upholding *The Code* (NMC, 2018b) at all times. This is an example of how UK legislation effects your practice as a nursing associate. Activity 5.3 helps you to explore these concepts further.

Activity 5.3   Critical thinking

Imagine that you are in the staff room at your place of work. This could be in any clinical setting – a hospital, community service, mental health unit or learning disability school. The topic of conversation is about marriage. Your colleagues are discussing the differences between marriage and civili partnership; no patients are mentioned in this debate. One group of perspectives is that there are no differences, whereas the alternative is that people who have civil partnerships are technically not married and people who have same-sex marriages have gay or lesbian weddings. Discuss the following questions with your supervisor or line manager:

1. What are the similarities between marriage and civil partnership?
2. Are people who have had a civil partnership married?
3. In this situation, how could you highlight that there is no such thing as a 'gay or lesbian wedding', in the same way that a wedding between a man and a woman would not be labelled as a 'straight wedding'?

An outline answer is available at the end of the chapter, but remember that every situation is different, so the answers discussed should not be used as rules – they provide direction for your reflective discussion with your supervisor or line manager.

Activity 5.3 encourages you to be a role model in the place where you work, thus upholding *The Code* (NMC, 2018b). Situations such as this are not easy, and it takes much courage to share an alternative perspective. The decision to act in this way links with the discussion in Chapter 1 about the 6Cs in *Leading Change, Adding Value* (NHS England, 2016). Remember that the person or people you are in a discussion with may not be aware of the legal difference, so by sharing this you are educating them. For more information about practice education, see Chapter 7. In Activity 5.3, although it is not directly about patient care, there is an extended link with inclusivity because you would be promoting inclusive behaviour of others. Read the next section to find out more about how to be inclusive regarding pregnancy and maternity.

7. Pregnancy and maternity

Throughout this book, the term 'patient' has been used to describe people who have health and social care needs, which includes terms such as 'service users' or 'clients' (you may hear some alternatives in clinical practice). However, we are now going to focus on anther protected characteristic from the Equality Act 2010, pregnancy and maternity. As briefly mentioned before, it is perfectly healthy to be pregnant, so a pregnant woman should not be referred to as a patient. With this in mind, for this section, the term 'pregnant woman' will be used in place of the term 'patient'.

As a nursing associate, your practice includes care across the lifespan of a person, which includes caring for women when they are pregnant, as well as their families (NMC, 2018a). Perhaps you have worked in a maternity setting before starting your apprenticeship, in which case caring for pregnant women will be familiar to you. However, many nursing associates have no experience of maternity care. It should be of some relief that caring for pregnant women has many similarities with caring for non-pregnant people. If you are apprehensive about caring for pregnant women, go back to Chapter 2 to revise your knowledge of acute and long-term person-centred care. The nursing process is directly relevant to caring for pregnant women; therefore, having worked in most other adult care settings, you will have developed transferable skills to care for pregnant women (Howatson-Jones et al., 2015). Much like other clinical environments you will have worked in, caring for pregnant women is a rewarding role. If you would like to read more about pregnancy and maternity care, see the annotated further reading section at the end of the chapter. For now, how do you ensure that your practice as a nursing associate in a pregnancy and maternity setting is person-centred?

As always, make sure you are competent and confident to meet the needs of pregnant women. In the majority of cases, pregnant women are well, and you may be required to teach them a skill such as breastfeeding (for more information on patient education, see Chapter 8), as well as completing routine health assessments, and you may be educating them about what happens at each stage of their pregnancy. You are not expected to have in-depth knowledge here, but signposting patients to valid and reliable information is within your scope of practice. Remember that if you are unsure of the answer to a question a woman asks, confidently let them know that you do not have that information, but you can ask their doctor or midwife to come and see them. This demonstrates that you understand the limits of your scope of practice, which will instil confidence in the pregnant woman.

Similar to other clinical environments, you may be required to care for the family and friends of pregnant women. Involving the women's family and/or friends as much as they would like is part of maternity care. Catering for specific family needs or wishes is also providing person-centred care. Think back to reading about religious beliefs in Chapters 4 and 5, and how we can honour those beliefs, where possible and appropriate, in clinical practice.

Unfortunately, pregnant women may be enduring what is known as pregnancy discrimination. The charity Maternity Action paraphrases the Equality Act 2010 definition of pregnancy discrimination as when a woman is treated unfairly because of her pregnancy; this could be termination of employment, not completing a pregnancy risk assessment, or preventing the promotion of a woman because they are pregnant (Maternity Action, 2019). It is likely that a woman or her family and friends may mention this while you are caring for her. Although you may not be able to take immediate action, you are able to identify options for the pregnant woman. Highlighting charitable services such as Maternity Action is one option, or the trust that you work for may have an in-house service for pregnant women. Take time to listen to her story and ask permission before sharing any personal information about her case with any service that your trust provides. It may be most appropriate for the pregnant woman to refer herself to the service, as this puts her in control of her situation; patient empowerment is an act of providing person-centred care (NMC, 2018b). Completing Activity 5.4 will enable you to explore how you can promote patient empowerment.

Activity 5.4   Critical thinking

Jo and Holly are a boyfriend and girlfriend who have recently found out that they are having a baby. Holly is ten weeks' pregnant and is feeling well. Jo is also healthy and six months ago started the transitioning process to living as a woman permanently; he has changed the spelling of his name from Joe to Jo. Jo and Holly have discussed their situation together and have agreed that they would like to continue their relationship. Jo is regularly seeing a therapist to help him transition to fully identifying as a woman, but at the moment he does not feel ready to identify fully and openly as a woman. Holly adamantly wants to support Jo but confides in you that she is worried for him, and she is concerned that the stress she feels will affect the baby.

What should you do in this situation? Discuss your answer with your supervisor or line manager.

An outline answer is available at the end of the chapter, but remember that every situation is different, so the answers discussed should not be used as rules – they provide direction for your reflective discussion with your supervisor or line manager.

Activity 5.4 is more complicated than others because Jo and Holly have more than one care need. In reality, this is more common; very rarely in clinical practice will you be caring for someone who has only one health or social care need. Discussing how to provide person-centred care in complex clinical situations with your supervisor or line manager will give you self-confidence and demonstrate that you are seeking to learn from others. The next section of this chapter focuses on race.

8. Race

Race can be defined as a patient's physical features, differing slightly to ethnicity, which can be described as someone's behaviour that is informed by heredity, ancestry or regional influences. In the Equality Act 2010, the term 'race' is used, but it includes someone's ethnic background. It is important to remember the differences between race and ethnicity to ensure that you are accurate in discussions with patients or colleagues, as well as in your documentation.

A patient's race is very personal and may be an important part of them as a person. You may hear patients speak of their family with reflective pride. One suggestion to ensure that you are providing person-centred care is to show a respectful and genuine interest in a patient's race, ethnicity or cultural heritage. You must ensure that you use your emotional intelligence in these situations to judge whether it is appropriate to discuss someone's racial background. Sometimes it may be an uncomfortable experience for the patient, in which case it should be avoided, but actively listening to a patient about their family's history may be a method to build trust and a rapport.

An important note to reiterate here is to never make presumptions. For example, if you are completing the admissions assessment for a patient and you assume that they are of a particular race, you may deeply offend them if you are incorrect. It is more appropriate to ask open questions. For example, if a question in the assessment pack requires the patient to identify their race, you could ask, 'How do you describe your race?' Asking the question in this way, you have made no assumptions and you have provided the patient with the opportunity to self-identify their race, thus respecting their individuality. This is another example of how to provide person-centred care and respect people's uniqueness. Read the next section to find out more about religion or belief as a protected characteristic.

9. Religion or belief

It is estimated that there are thousands of different religions around the world, although most people can only list the most commonly known ones. Furthermore, within each religion, there could be several denominations, which are variant ways of practising the religion. Similar to race, religion can be an integral part of a patient's life. If so, religion may influence the patient's decision-making, and – providing they have mental capacity, are legally an adult, and meet the four criteria of informed consent – you may be required to adapt your care to meet their needs. This means being able to make reasonable adjustments where possible.

Religion was briefly discussed in Chapter 4 in the context of palliative and end of life care. At this point, consider going back to Chapter 4 to reread the sections specifically on religion to refresh your memory on some religious practices regarding end of life care. For now, what does it mean to be able to make reasonable adjustments in your practice to cater for a patient's religious needs? First, it involves having a conversation with the patient for whom you are caring. Ask the patient if they have any specific needs relating to their religion that you should be aware of (e.g. the patient may be Muslim and choose to eat halal food). Questions such as these are important to ask when admitting the patient or when you are first meeting them, to ensure that they are made to feel as comfortable as possible. However, in some circumstances, the patient may not be able to answer your questions. In such circumstances, with informed consent from the patient, speak with their family, friends or religious leader to discuss if the patient has any specific requirements. Sometimes you may not be able to gain informed consent from the patient, if they do not speak English, for example. Requesting an interpreter is the most reliable course of action here; do not ask a family member or friend to translate as they are not impartial to the patient's care.

A challenging question to ask yourself is: When does a reasonable adjustment become unreasonable? This is a difficult mark to measure. Every situation in clinical practice is different, so there is no fixed rule about what is a reasonable adjustment or not. Some thoughts for guidance are: Does the request impact negatively on other patients? For example, a patient may request to be in a side room of a ward, but if there is a patient who has a contagious infection on the ward they will need to be in the side room to mitigate the risk of the infection spreading. In such circumstances, it is an unreasonable adjustment to move the patient in the multiple bedded section of the ward to a side room. However, if a patient has had three consecutive nights of no sleep due to the noise in the ward and there is a spare side room, it could be a reasonable adjustment to make. In any of these circumstances, always check with your supervisor or line manager before taking action to check that your decision does not have an impact on other patients in the environment you are working in, which you may not be aware of. Lastly, if a patient's request cannot be carried out, explain to the patient and their family and friends the rationale as to why, remembering to maintain the confidentiality of others at all times.

At this point, we have considered all of the protected characteristics in the Equality Act 2010, as well as providing you with some suggestions of how to promote inclusivity in your practice, therefore ensuring that you are providing person-centred care. However, this chapter is to be used as a resource to signpost you to other content and literature. With this in mind, make sure that you consistently consider how to be more inclusive in your clinical practice as a nursing associate, as well as challenging yourself to find more ways of adopting a person-centred approach.

Chapter summary

Inclusivity is integral to person-centred care. In other words, to provide person-centred care as a nursing associate is to be inclusive. Being able to recognise people's individuality and adapt your practice to meet their specific needs demonstrates inclusivity. Adapting your practice is known as making a reasonable adjustment, and you can work collaborative with the MDT and the patient's family, friends and carers to identify what constitutes a reasonable adjustment. Remember to ensure that you reflect on your practice, as this process will help you to identify significant learning points about how to enhance inclusivity in your practice. Have the confidence to seek feedback from colleagues too, because they may have noticed things that you have done well or could improve on, which you did not see. In return, support them in developing their reflective practice too. Working together as an effective team will ultimately improve the standards of inclusive person-centred care even further. Proactively learn from senior and experienced colleagues too. Most people in the MDT are willing to share their knowledge, and this is to your benefit, as well as the benefit of the patients you care for. Lastly, ensure that reflective discussions and feedback take place in an appropriate location within the clinical setting, perhaps the staff room, the hospital library, or a designated learning and teaching place.

Activities: Brief outline answers

Activity 5.1 Critical thinking (page 73)

The Equality Act 2010 is integral to your practice as a nursing associate. One way that you could answer this question is by noting the platforms of the *Standards of Proficiency for Nursing Associates* (NMC, 2018a) that are linked with this chapter:

- *Platform 1: Being an accountable professional.* As a practitioner on a professional register, you have ownership of your conduct in clinical practice and you are accountable to the NMC. In relation to inclusivity, you are empowered to take responsibility for your own professional development and quality assurance, which can be achieved by using reflective practice and seeking feedback from colleagues and patients.
- *Platform 3: Provide and monitor care.* Your clinical practice focuses on a holistic perspective (see Chapter 1). Therefore, as a nursing associate, you are able to identify specific care needs for each patient, as well as their family, friends and carers, and provide them with bespoke evidence-based care that meets their needs. This may involve making reasonable adjustments, and as an important member of the MDT you are able to communicate that with all of the professionals in the team you are a part of.
- *Platform 4: Working in teams.* Not only do you practise with integrity and inclusivity, but you are a role model to other members of staff. As you spend a significant amount of your time with patients, you are able to contribute to team reflections and advocate the needs of the patients you are caring for. Maintaining effective communication among the MDT is paramount in order for the patient to receive person-centred care, and nursing associates have an integral role in this process.

Activity 5.2 Critical thinking (page 74)

Legally, Raheel is an adult, so he should be admitted to the adult ward. His parents have requested for him to be admitted to the paediatric ward as they may have better facilities to meet Raheel's autism. If there is the bed space and the ward manager is happy, this request may be accommodated. However, it is more than likely that Raheel will need to be admitted to the adult ward. At this point, you could explain to the parents that your training and scope of practice includes all four specialisms of nursing, including the care of people with additional learning needs. Once you have answered any of their questions (or found answers by asking a senior colleague), the parents' anxieties will have reduced. The salient learning point for this activity is that good care is not totally dependent on the environment, but the practitioners providing the care. This is another example of the important contribution you can make to the MDT and the provision of person-centred care.

Activity 5.3 Critical thinking (page 77)

1. *What are the similarities between marriage and civil partnership?* The similarities are that both ceremonies are a legal recognition of a relationship between two people. People can apply for a mortgage together as, for example, husband and wife, husband and husband, or wife and wife. For more details of the similarities, see the Citizens Advice web page in the annotated further reading section at the end of the chapter.

2. *Are people who have had a civil partnership married?* Technically, people who have had a civil partnership are not married, as this is a different ceremony. However, it should be noted that many people believe the differences are so minimal that they may refer to their partner as their husband or wife, regardless of whether they had a marriage or a civil partnership.

3. *In this situation, how could you highlight that there is no such thing as a 'gay or lesbian wedding', in the same way that a wedding between a man and a woman would not be labelled as a 'straight wedding'?* One way that you could politely challenge this view is to share the facts about the situation; this should be done with calm and with respect for the alternative point of view. You may mention that there is no legal difference between a marriage of two people of either the same or opposite gender; therefore, their marital ceremony is a wedding regardless of their sex or sexual orientation. Remember to present this information in a way that cannot be misinterpreted as dismissive of another point of view; you may start by saying, 'Have you considered …?' Use your common sense and emotional intelligence to judge what is appropriate in any situation to ensure that you uphold the values of *The Code* (NMC, 2018b).

Activity 5.4 Critical thinking (page 78)

There is no gold standard answer to Jo and Holly's situation. However, start by actively listening to Holly's concerns and show her that you are genuinely empathetic of her circumstances. Point out that although you are not a specialist, you can be an impartial person to listen to her story. You could then suggest specialist services that Holly and Jo could be referred to for additional support during her pregnancy. Remember to follow the care plan for Holly and objectively document the person-centred care you provided, as well as the findings of your holistic assessment.

Annotated further reading

Citizens Advice (2020) *Living Together, Marriage and Civil Partnership*. Available at: www.citizensadvice.org.uk/family/living-together-marriage-and-civil-partnership/

This web page will provide you with clear explanations of the legal differences and similarities between marriage and civil partnership.

Equality and Human Rights Commission (2019) *Equality Act Guidance*. Available at: www.equalityhumanrights.com/en/advice-and-guidance/equality-act-guidance

The information on this web page is a very comprehensive guidance on the Equality Act 2010. Helpfully, it is broken down into smaller subsections, so you do not need to read a huge document from cover to cover – you can pick and choose what information you need to read to develop your knowledge.

GOV.UK (2020) *Definition of Disability Under the Equality Act 2010*. Available at: www.gov.uk/definition-of-disability-under-equality-act-2010

Use this web page to read more about the definition of disability in relation to the Equality Act 2010. There are other links that you can access via this web page that will develop your wider understanding of disability, discrimination and the Equality Act 2010.

Royal College of Nursing (RCN) (2016) *Equality, Diversity and Rights*. Available at: https://rcni.com/hosted-content/rcn/first-steps/equality-diversity-and-rights

The Royal College of Nursing has a number of very useful articles, short in length, about inclusivity, anti-discriminatory practice, reasonable adjustments and many other related topics. Follow the link to read more about the suggestions made in this chapter, as well as other recommendations made by the Royal College of Nursing. For your next appraisal, consider reading and reflecting on the articles listed on this web page if you would like to know more about how to promote inclusivity in your clinical practice as a nursing associate.

Royal College of Nursing (RCN) (2019) *Nurses in Maternity Care: RCN Report*. Available at: www.rcn.org.uk/professional-development/publications/pub-007640

This document is not a competency checklist, like the *Standards of Proficiency for Nursing Associates* (NMC, 2018a), but it provides commentary of the knowledge and skills that nurses and nursing associates require to work in a maternity setting. In the report, advice is also provided about how to shape your CPD when working in a maternity environment. Remember to always read and follow the local trust policy that you are working in.

Skills for Health (2019) *Resources*. Available at: www.skillsforhealth.org.uk/resources

Skills for Health is a not-for-profit organisation that works to develop and improve the UK healthcare workforce. This link will take you to their web page of resources, which cover a broad range of topics, including lots of material related to inclusivity and person-centred care.

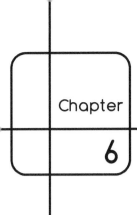

Chapter 6

Public health

NMC STANDARDS OF PROFICIENCY FOR NURSING ASSOCIATES

This chapter will address the following platforms and proficiencies:

Platform 1: Being an accountable professional

At the point of registration, the nursing associate will be able to:

1.7 describe the principles of research and how research findings are used to inform evidence-based practice

Platform 2: Promoting health and preventing ill health

At the point of registration, the nursing associate will be able to:

2.3 describe the principles of epidemiology, demography, and genomics and how these may influence health and wellbeing outcomes
2.4 understand the factors that may lead to inequalities in health outcomes
2.5 understand the importance of early years and childhood experiences and the possible impact on life choices, mental, physical and behavioural health and wellbeing
2.6 understand and explain the contribution of social influences, health literacy, individual circumstances, behaviours and lifestyle choices to mental, physical and behavioural health outcomes
2.8 promote health and prevent ill health by understanding the evidence base for immunisation, vaccination and herd immunity

Introduction

In Chapter 2, the assessment and management of acute and long-term conditions were discussed. Being able to provide person-centred care to patients who are unwell is a primary aim of your practice as a nursing associate. However, what if you could support patients to reduce the risk of them becoming unwell? This would save the NHS money, as well as empowering patients to live independently with their family, friends and carers. In this chapter, we are going to explore your role in public health, a speciality that focuses on promoting health and wellbeing to enable everyone to have healthy lives. Public health is an intrinsic part of your scope of practice and will contribute to preventing patients becoming unwell or deteriorating. To do this, you need to understand the influencing factors of patients' health. There are countless influences on each person's health, but in this chapter you will learn how to focus your critical thinking skills to understand the social determinants of health. Understanding the influence of the social determinants of health will enable you to provide bespoke care that promotes positive impacts for patients. Furthermore, we are going to explore health inequalities, understanding why people living in some areas are healthier than others and what can be done to create equality of health. In summary, the content of this chapter is integral to your practice as a nursing associate, and will enable you to contribute to the health and wellbeing of people in your care, as well as their family, friends and carers.

Public health

Before defining public health, pause for a moment and consider the phrase 'good health'. Promoting people's health is a common thread throughout all of the chapters of this book, but how do we know what optimum health is? Most people could describe, in their own way, what they think and feel good health is (e.g. referring back to a time in their life when they felt the healthiest). Most people reflect on their youth as the period when they were most healthy, sharing anecdotes of having lots of energy and feeling fit. However, if we pull on this thread, does everyone describe good health in the same way?

Everyone's interpretation of good health is **subjective**. In other words, they have a personal opinion of what good health means to them. With this in mind, you need to take the time to identify what constitutes good health for each patient you are caring for. Without this knowledge, you are unable to provide person-centred care because you do not know what the patient's good health goal looks like. Think back to the nursing process discussed in Chapter 1 – the second stage of the process is patient goals (Howatson-Jones et al., 2015). We discussed how each patient will have different goals because they have different interpretations of good health. For example, a primary school teacher may want to be healthy enough to return to work, whereas a retired schoolteacher may want to feel healthy enough to be discharged to their home rather than to a rehabilitation ward. These examples demonstrate that there are similarities between many people, but their perception of good health is personal. Before moving on to read more about what public health is, remember that good health is not limited to physical health. Patients may also aspire to improve their psychological (possibly socio-economic, spiritual or religious) health, so always ensure that the first stage of the nursing process – your assessment – is person-centred (Howatson-Jones et al., 2015).

Public health is a broad speciality, where improving and protecting people's health (physical, psychological or other) is the priority (Health Careers, 2020). Public health is dynamic because some interventions aim to promote and protect the good health of individual people, whereas other interventions involve improving the health of a group of people. Clearly identifying which group of people is important to ensure that the intervention is bespoke and meets their needs (much like when you complete a person-centred assessment, but for a group of people). One group of people may live in a certain area and have similar ethnic backgrounds or the same learning disability. But how does a public health initiative work, and how does public health relate to your practice as a nursing associate?

Public health is relevant to people across their lifespan, from conception to death. Therefore, public health is directly relevant to your practice as a nursing associate because your scope of practice includes caring for people throughout their lifespan. Throughout a person's life, public health initiatives aim to identify how the health of people in different communities can be improved and protected. They do this first by researching **health risks** and calculating the probable severity of health risks to different groups of people who are living in different areas and at different points in their lifespan. Identifying these risks and the people who are most at risk of becoming unwell or deteriorating informs public health plans to mitigate these health risks (i.e. protecting people's health). Public health also involves researching the impact of socio-economic and environmental influences of health (see the discussion of the Marmot Reviews later in this chapter). According to Health Careers (2020), there are three priorities of public health: preventing disease, prolonging life and promoting health.

The **incidence** of infectious diseases across the world causes many preventable deaths each year, but public health initiatives can save lives. Vaccinations, for example, significantly reduce the health risks of certain diseases, which is why vaccinations are a public health initiative to prevent disease (for more information about vaccinations, immunisation and herd immunity, see later in this chapter).

Prolonging life can be achieved by using research results and findings to identify which people are vulnerable to health risks, then educating people how to reduce these risks. For example, women who have been through their menopause are at risk of their bones becoming weak, a condition called **osteoporosis** (also colloquially known as brittle bone disease). This is because a reduced level of the hormone **oestrogen** leads to an increase in bone reabsorption. Women who have an early menopause or have their ovaries removed are more at risk of osteoporosis because they have a longer period of time throughout their lifespan of reduced oestrogen levels, and hence greater bone reabsorption. However, public health initiatives educate women and empower them to reduce the risk of osteoporosis via regular exercise, smoking cessation, maintaining low levels of alcohol consumption, and eating a balanced diet rich in calcium and vitamin D (Royal Osteoporosis Society, 2020). Making these positive lifestyle choices reduces the risk of osteoporosis and the risk of breaking bones, particularly major breaks such as the femur or cranium, which prolongs healthy life.

Public health also involves promoting a healthy lifestyle, which ultimately reduces the **prevalence** of acute and long-term conditions. Reducing the prevalence of disease reduces public dependency on the NHS, therefore saving money, which can be redirected to support underfunded health and social care services. Furthermore, reducing the risk of illness contributes to people living long, healthy lives, both physically and psychologically. Public health is an inclusive discipline that focuses on improving and protecting the lives of individuals and communities. Activity 6.1 will help you to consolidate your understanding of public health.

Activity 6.1   Research

This activity has two parts:

1. Watch the following video and summarise the key components of public health: **https:// youtu.be/oy1CAMObRzc**
2. Define the following important public health terms using the information on the following web page: **www.healthcareers.nhs.uk/working-health/working-public-health/what-public-health**

    *   wellbeing;
    *   population health;
    *   health inequalities;
    *   social determinants of health.

An outline answer is provided at the end of the chapter.

You now have a consolidated definition of what public health is and its positive impact for patients. Furthermore, we have discussed why public health is integral to your practice as a nursing associate. The next section of the chapter looks at Public Health England (PHE), an organisation focused on and committed to public health practice.

PHE was established in 2013 as an executive constituent of the Department of Health and Social Care (DHSC, formerly the Department of Health). It houses researchers and practitioners who specialise in public health, who were previously spread across the country. It has a mandate to improve and protect the health of the population in England; the devolved states of the UK have similar public health agencies: Public Health Scotland, Public Health Wales and Public Health Agency (Northern Ireland). PHE also aims to reduce health inequalities, particularly by supporting people who are disadvantaged. It works towards its aims by investing in public health research at the national level and collaborating with local government. Focusing on working with local government enables bespoke funding to be provided to meet the public health needs of the communities within the local government remit. Furthermore, public health specialists work with local government to advise them how to protect and promote the good health of the communities they serve. PHE regularly evaluates its initiatives through research, ensuring its practice is consistently evidence-based. It produces important resources about public health that are relevant to your practice as a nursing associate. Activity 6.2 will help to ensure that you keep up to date.

Activity 6.2   Research

In Activity 3.5 in Chapter 3, it was suggested that you subscribe to GOVUK email alerts to ensure that you receive up-to-date information from the Department of Health and Social Care (DHSC). However, reading emails may not be ideal for you. An alternative for ensuring that you are kept up to date with PHE is to subscribe to its YouTube channel: **www.youtube.com/ user/publichealthengland**

It is important to note that not all of the important information you need is disseminated via YouTube, but some of the material you need to be aware of may be communicated in video form. Other YouTube channels may similarly have valuable information presented in an easily accessible way. However, if viewing this material, you should exercise the highest level of caution and critical thinking. While some information may be valid and reliable, YouTube is a platform that does not have the rigorous peer-review process that academic journals have. In other words, anyone can post material on YouTube that may be factually inaccurate, or even dangerous. Similarly, the website Wikipedia is an open publishing platform. With this in mind, always ensure that you cross-check the information you read or view anywhere online with a valid and reliable source.

For this activity, visit the PHE YouTube channel and watch a video that interests you or is relevant to your area of clinical practice. Discuss with your supervisor or line manager how you could disseminate the information in the video among your team, as well as how using the PHE YouTube channel could support reflective development.

As this activity is based on your own reflection, there is no outline answer provided at the end of the chapter.

Social determinants of health

In Chapter 1, there was an 'Understanding the theory' box that introduced the social determinants of health. In this section of the chapter, we are going to explore the social determinants of health in more detail. First, though, we will recap what the social determinants of health are about.

The most recognised publication about the social determinants of health is the Dahlgren-Whitehead rainbow, which illustrates the social determinants of health listed in the aforementioned 'Understanding the theory' box in Chapter 1. The rainbow has been published in many forms, but one of the most recent is in a World Health Organization (WHO) strategy about reducing the social inequality of health in Europe (Dahlgren and Whitehead, 2006). The Dahlgren-Whitehead rainbow is a useful way to present the interconnection of different social determinants of health; however, any social science discipline is complex and challenging to define. Taking this into account, remember that the Dahlgren-Whitehead rainbow is a representation of a complex social system and may not be an exact representation of every patient's determinants of health. For example, the living and working condition 'unemployment' suggests that a period of unemployment has a negative impact on someone's health. In reality, there are many people who have had periods of unemployment, for a variety of reasons, that have healthy lifestyles. In other words, use the Dahlgren-Whitehead rainbow as a guide but be led by your person-centred assessment of the patient.

Genomics and the social determinants of health

Determinants of health are not only social constructs. **Genetics** has a significant influence on people's health too. Genetics can be described as what is inherited from biological parents. A patient's genome is the inherited characteristics specific to them; **genomics** is the study of the genome. You inherit many characteristics from your biological parents: physical appearance, personality traits and long-term conditions. One part of genomics is to calculate the probability of inheriting certain characteristics from your parents, as each characteristic of your biological parents is not guaranteed to be passed down to you. For example, if your parents both have brown eyes, it is not 100 per cent guaranteed that you will have brown eyes too; the likely colour of your eyes can be calculated depending on your parents' **genome**. Understanding the probability of children inheriting long-term conditions is important for reducing their likelihood, which involves making positive lifestyle choices that reduce the influence of the social determinants of health. In other words, your health is affected by both your genetics and social determinants.

Diabetes is a common long-term condition that many of the patients you care for will have. Genomics and the social determinants of health can be used to explain the increase in the prevalence of diabetes in some areas throughout the last few decades. From a genomic perspective, the likelihood of a person inheriting Type 1 diabetes is determined by one or both of the biological parents of a child having a **dominant gene** in their **deoxyribonucleic acid** (DNA). A dominant gene means that they have the disease and their children also have a significant chance of growing up with Type 1 diabetes. Another set of biological parents may be carriers of the condition (i.e. they have a **recessive gene** in their DNA). In this case, the biological parents do not have the long-term condition, but their children (or in some cases their grandchildren) are significantly likely to grow up with Type 1 diabetes. These likelihoods are calculated through genetic testing to identify how active a dominant or recessive gene is. However, this likelihood may not be 100 per cent accurate because social determinants of health also affect the likelihood of developing long-term conditions.

Type 1 diabetes is most commonly inherited and develops in childhood, although not in all cases (e.g. Theresa May, the former Prime Minister of the UK, was diagnosed with Type 1 diabetes in her fifties). However, Type 2 diabetes usually develops from the age of 40 years onwards (although again, not in all cases). If a person's parents have Type 2 diabetes, there is an increased chance of inheriting the long-term condition, although the social determinants of health have a greater effect. Referring back to the Dahlgren-Whitehead rainbow, food is a lifestyle factor in determining health. Consistent consumption of fatty, sugary and carbohydrate-rich food increases insulin production from the pancreas to control capillary blood glucose (CBG) levels in the blood. Too much sugar causes blood to become very sticky, and hence it can clot and/or cause damage to capillaries. Over time, it is common for people living with Type 2 diabetes to develop insulin resistance, which means that despite insulin being produced by the pancreas, the cells are unable to process it as a source of energy. As a result, patients need to control their sugar levels by adopting positive lifestyle choices for their diet, or eventually become dependent on medicated control of insulin – this is known as Type 2 diabetes. This description is an example of how the social determinants of health can be the main factor in developing long-term conditions. However, it is important to note that this description is not the only eventuality. As previously discussed, there are multiple factors of health, and these examples are used to explain how genomics and the social determinants of health both affect health. As a nursing associate, you need to be able to understand the interrelation of both explanations to be able to educate patients in your care about how to reduce the risk of developing long-term conditions and protect their good health. Read the next section to link what you have learned so far in this chapter with the 100,000 Genomes Project, led by Genomics England. This section of the chapter will directly relate to Chapter 8 and your future practice as a nursing associate.

Originally, scientists wanted to be able to read all of the genetic codes in a genome, as this would enable them to know what long-term conditions a patient is likely to develop. This was first achieved in the middle of the twentieth century – it took 13 years and cost £2 billion. However, as technology has developed, reading a genetic code can be sequenced within a day and costs around £1,000 (HEE, 2014). Modern technology has enabled Genomics England to establish their 100,000 Genomes Project – the sequencing of 100,000 genomes of patients with rare long-term conditions or cancer. This project provides valuable information about diseases at the genetic level, and hence scientists have the knowledge to provide more personalised healthcare (for more information about personalised medicine, see Chapter 8).

Genomics will be pivotal in the provision of person-centred care during the twenty-first century, and the future of genomics will be revisited in Chapter 8. For now, see the useful websites section at the end of the chapter for a link to an excellent website provided by Health Education England's Genomics Education Programme. Here, you will find a wide variety of material to learn more about genomics, as well as how you can support patients who are undergoing genetic therapy.

Now that you have developed an understanding of genomics and the social determinants of health, you can begin to apply this knowledge to your practice as a nursing associate. Read the next section of this chapter to learn more about how to promote healthy early years and childhood development to increase the chances of a happy and healthy life in adulthood.

Early years and childhood development

The key stages in the human lifespan were outlined in Chapter 1. In the context of this chapter, early years and childhood development are fundamental to the child growing up and having a healthy adult life. Arguably, childhood is one of the most important stages of the lifespan for public health initiatives because it provides an opportunity to significantly reduce health risks for the majority of someone's lifespan. According to the WHO (2018), public health for children can reduce the prevalence of physical and psychological conditions – obesity, coronary heart disease and mental health conditions are some examples. Furthermore, there can be additional positive impacts of effective public health initiatives for children's health, including wider socio-economic influences on increased health literacy (for more information, see later in this chapter), numeracy, a reduction in criminal activity, and greater financial income (Irwin et al., 2007). Your practice as a nursing associate includes caring for children, so how can you promote and protect good health and wellbeing for children?

The WHO commissioned a project to collect evidence from successful public health initiatives for children around the world and published their findings in a report (Irwin et al., 2007). The report focuses on children aged from birth to 8 years, and the key findings were:

- a holistic approach to childhood development is required for effective and healthy childhood development;
- a positive environment nurtured by parents, guardians or caregivers, supported by local, regional, national and international organisations, enables healthy childhood development;
- it is important for all parents and caregivers, educators, local authorities, and governments to recognise their responsibilities in providing a healthy start to a child's life, as their actions determine the success of early years and childhood development, which leads to healthy adulthood;
- socio-economic and health inequalities should be investigated and reduced to enable every child to have a healthy development.

The key findings listed here summarise a lengthy document – this is high-level guidance. Your role as a nursing associate is to apply findings such as these to your practice. For example, one of the findings is that parents and caregivers (guardians) have a huge influence in positive childhood development, which is why one of your roles is to support parents/caregivers to provide a nurturing environment for the child to grow up in. This could involve ensuring that parents/caregivers have access to information about schools or can afford healthy food on a budget. Although you may not give parents/caregivers direct advice yourself, you can signpost them to reliable sources of information. Always remember to ensure that you document your practice clearly and involve your supervisor.

Health inequalities

So far in this chapter, the social determinants of health and genetics have been discussed in relation to public health – promoting and protecting good health. An important question to ask is: Why do some individuals and communities have better health in comparison to others? These differences are known as health inequalities, which can be defined as preventable differences in physical and psychological health between people in society (Williams et al., 2020). Health inequalities also include the differing influences of health (e.g. access to appropriate health or social care, poorer standards of housing, limited number of healthy food choices). In other words, health inequalities are collectively known as unfair, avoidable differences in the social determinants of health that are detrimental to health.

According to the King's Fund, there are four common health inequality categories, which are listed below with some examples:

- socio-economic background (e.g. job security and reliable income);
- geographic background (e.g. living in a city or the countryside);
- protected characteristics (e.g. ethnicity or gender – for more information, see Chapter 5);
- social exclusion (e.g. the homeless or people living with alcohol misuse).

(Williams et al., 2020)

If people are associated with one of these categories, it does not mean they have poorer health. For example, a person who lives in a social housing block does not necessarily have worse health in comparison to someone who lives in a detached house in the suburbs. However, the results from public health research statistically demonstrate that people are more likely to experience health inequalities if they are linked with one or more of these categories. As a result, physical and psychological long-term conditions are more likely to develop, and their life expectancy is shorter in comparison to people who do not experience health inequalities. With this in mind, what can you do as a nursing associate to reduce health inequalities and provide person-centred care?

Health literacy

Literacy is the ability to read and write; however, health literacy is not limited to being able to comprehend literature about acute and long-term conditions. Health literacy is the ability, availability and motivation to understand health-related information and apply this to positive lifestyle choices to promote and protect health (WHO, 2009). Evidently, good health literacy can improve and maintain the good health of patients, as well as their families, friends and carers. However, poor health literacy can be a health inequality, meaning that the opportunity for people to adopt positive behaviours towards their health can be limited.

Clearly, there are many influencing factors that determine a person's health literacy. For example, not being able to read health information can be limiting, especially if the patient is not confident reading English, has an additional learning need, or is blind. Furthermore, if the information is written with complexity, people reading the information may be prevented from understanding the key messages. Approximately 60 per cent of people in the UK have a disadvantaged health literacy when reading health literature containing statistics because the information is not presented in an accessible way (NHS Digital Service Manual, 2019).

It is important to note that no one is deliberately publishing information with the intent to exclude people. Health literacy is about thinking how to be more inclusive when publishing information for the public to read or view. In other words, when producing or sharing information, it is important to ensure that the material is accessible. This is evidence of how health literacy is part of your scope of practice as a nursing associate providing person-centred care.

The NHS has developed nine principles to guide professionals in how to produce health information material that meets the standards of the NHS Constitution (NHS Design Service Manual, 2018, 2019). As a nursing associate, you may be involved in producing some educational material for patients, but more likely you will be disseminating information about a patient's condition to them and their family, friends and carers. Before doing so, you can use your critical thinking skills to assess if the information meets the needs of the patient before giving it to them by asking questions related to the nine design principles from the NHS. Some examples are listed below:

- Is the information person-centred?
- Does the information meet the patient's needs?
- Is the information inclusive and representative?
- Can the information be applied to the patient's wider circumstances?

These questions are only suggestions. You can adapt them to be more appropriate to the clinical environment and situations you work in.

So far in this chapter, we have explored the interrelation of the social determinants of health, health inequalities and health literacy. These three concepts affect the lifestyle choices people make, which by extension influences people's physical and psychological health. But what evidence is there that this is happening? Furthermore, how can you find out more about these concepts in the area you work in? To answer these questions, you need to read The Marmot Reviews.

The Marmot Reviews

As discussed so far in this chapter, health inequalities and health literacy have a huge impact on how healthy people are, not forgetting the social determinants of health and genetic factors too. In 2010, Sir Michael Marmot published an extensive review of health inequalities in England called *Fair Society Healthy Lives* (Marmot et al., 2010). This was the first national collation of evidence and analysis of health inequalities. The findings were deeply shocking and confirmed the worst predictions.

Until this point in time, the success and development of a country was measured by economic growth. It was advocated in the Marmot Review that equality of health and wellbeing for the whole population should be included in the measurement of a country's sustainable development. An assessment was made of the health inequalities in England at the time. The difference between good and poor health was identified as having a significantly steep gradient caused by social inequality. In other words, the less a person's social status, the worse their health. This may appear obvious, but how severely a person's health was affected was still unknown. One shocking statistic was that a huge number of people could be living longer if there was more social and health equity. The collective total of how many extra years people could have lived was calculated between 1.3 and 2.5 million. The scale of health inequality was cause for alarm, and hence the Marmot Review included many recommendations to reduce the negative impact that health inequality was having on the public.

The overarching recommendation of the Marmot Review was reducing health inequalities, which is of national importance for society. However, limiting public health initiatives to support only those with low socio-economic backgrounds is short-sighted and would be ineffective in balancing health inequalities. All public health initiatives should be inclusive and proportionate to the severity of health impairment – from national government to local authorities. Most importantly, public health initiatives should empower families and individuals to have ownership of their health, as well as being supported in making positive lifestyle choices. Although nursing associates were not created in 2010, this recommendation is relevant to your scope of practice today – hence the importance of your role in public health. The Marmot Review highlighted that reducing health inequalities would have widespread benefits for society as a whole, both for the economy and for individuals living a longer, more fulfilling life. Many government frameworks and local policies were established to meet the recommendations of the Marmot Review. In 2020, a ten-year review was published to evaluate the impact.

The review of the first review of health inequalities was called *Health Equity in England* (Marmot et al., 2020). This review included very interesting findings in comparison with the first review. First, health inequalities are still undoubtably caused by the social determinants of health. However, the life expectancy of people living in England has plateaued for the first time in 100 years, a finding that is concerning. Although it is positive that people are not living shorter lives, no improvement in health is an indicator that the improvement of society has stalled. This strengthens the evidence that the social determinants of health have a significant impact on health inequalities. Another finding of this review is that more people are living greater amounts of their lives in ill health. The cost of this to the NHS and the economy has increased, resulting in some services being underfunded. Limiting the finances of services that improve the social determinants of health further catalyses health inequalities, making the overall situation much worse. However, there were some positive findings.

Despite widespread funding limitations, some local authorities have developed a number of evidence-based public health interventions that have reduced some health inequalities in their communities. This suggests that bespoke, locally driven public health initiatives which are person-centred are most effective. It is emphasised in this review that the health inequalities present in England are still preventable, which is why the recommendations of the first review were updated.

Recommendations for the next decade include the establishment of a national health inequality strategy, as well as balancing the inequality of health between the North and South of England. You can read more of the recommendations made in the review by accessing the report, listed in the annotated further reading section at the end of the chapter. It is important to note that evidence from this review suggests that local public health initiatives are most effective in reducing health inequalities, which results in many socio-economic benefits for everyone. With this in mind, what can you do as a nursing associate to support the national drive to balance health inequalities? Read the next section of this chapter for one example.

How to promote health

There are many ways to promote the health of patients and their family, friends and carers. Practice education is an important part of your role as a nursing associate, especially in providing person-centred care. If patients have a comprehensive understanding of their health, they will be empowered to have ownership of protecting and promoting good health. This meets one of the recommendations of *Health Equity in England* (Marmot et al., 2020). Chapter 7 focuses on practice education, but in this chapter we are going to discuss how immunisations, vaccinations and herd immunity promote and protect good health.

First, we need to define the difference between immunisation and vaccination. Immunisation is when your body has the natural defences against an infection or disease (i.e. you are immune), whereas a vaccination is an administration of a vaccine that stimulates your body to have immunity against an infection or disease (PHE, 2018a). An example of having immunity is when you develop symptoms of the common cold and after a few days are fully recovered. An example of a disease prevented by a vaccine is measles. Immunisation and vaccinations are evidently linked with public health because they are about protecting people from illnesses. Most vaccines are administered during childhood, hence why public health is so important for children and young people. There is a list of all licensed vaccines in the UK, as well as at what age they should be administered. This document is called *The Green Book* (PHE, 2014); you can find a link to it in the annotated further reading section at the end of the chapter. If you are involved in immunisations and vaccinations, it is imperative that you read this document to protect the safety and wellbeing of the patients you are caring for. For example, there are different types of vaccines, and some types cannot be administered to people who have **immunodeficiency**.

Some people choose not to have vaccines. This could be for religious or cultural reasons, but as long as the person has mental capacity this is their choice. Vaccinations can be an ethical consideration for some, such as a concern for animal welfare (some vaccines are produced containing animal products). Choosing not to have a vaccine increases the risk of an individual catching a disease. However, if too many people are not vaccinated, there can be a disease outbreak. The high transmission of a disease within a community is known as an **epidemic**, and if the disease spreads across a whole country or continent, or around the world, a **pandemic** is declared by the WHO. The medical practice of **epidemiology** is the study of how a disease is transmitted during an epidemic or pandemic, as well as potential methods to control the spread of disease. The Covid-19 pandemic is a good example of how an epidemic developed very quickly into a pandemic. The severity of the Covid-19 pandemic was caused by a number of factors, predominantly because no one had immunity. Vaccinations, however, are a way to control the transmission of diseases.

PHE monitors how many people are vaccinated against certain diseases, as this figure determines **herd immunity**. Herd immunity is the sufficient number of people in a population vaccinated against a disease (or who have natural immunity through previous exposure to the disease) that sufficiently protects the non-vaccinated members of the population. In other words, herd immunity means that the risk of an epidemic or pandemic is significantly reduced for that disease. As a nursing associate, you may be involved in administering vaccinations or educating patients about the vaccinations they or their child are having.

Remember that vaccinations and immunisations are not the only way you can protect and promote patients' health; this has been used as one example for the purposes of this chapter. There are many other ways you can adopt public health practice as a nursing associate. Always remember to adhere to your local trust's policy and regularly meet with your supervisor or line manager to discuss how you can improve and enhance your practice.

Chapter summary

Public health is fundamental to your role as a nursing associate. While caring for patients who are physically or psychologically unwell is important, promoting their health and wellbeing empowers patients to live longer, healthier and more fulfilling lives. Determining the goals of patient health should always involve the patient and their family, friends and carers. Thus, including patients in the nursing process (see Chapter 1) is one way to provide person-centred care. To support patients in making positive lifestyle choices requires you to understand their social determinants of health. Understanding the background to patients' health can be on an individual level or for a whole community. However, remember that the social determinants of health are not the only

(Continued)

(Continued)

influences of health. The science of genomics has enabled precise diagnoses of acute illness and the likelihood of developing long-term conditions. If patients choose to learn more about this, they can make positive lifestyle choices earlier, therefore promoting and protecting their health and wellbeing. Public health is also about reducing health inequalities. Some communities have disproportionate poorer health outcomes, but your public health practice as a nursing associate can contribute to reducing these inequalities. Make sure that you keep up to date with new research and evidence related to public health. For advice on how to keep your practice current, see Chapter 8.

Activities: Brief outline answers

Activity 6.1 Research (page 88)

1. The video emphasises the three key components of public health: preventing disease, prolonging life and promoting health. Remember that there are alternative definitions of public health, and your local trust may emphasise a slightly different public health strategy. This is because each trust serves their local community or specific areas of health and social care. Your trust may be a major trauma unit or neurological centre, for instance. With this in mind, it is important for you to understand local trust policy and how to ensure that your practice adheres to it. Discuss these points with your supervisor or line manager.

2. The answer to this question can be found in a drop-down menu about public health terms:

    *   *Wellbeing*: A positive physical and psychological state.
    *   *Population health*: The health and influencing factors of health across a whole population.
    *   *Health inequalities*: Preventable disadvantages of health and wellbeing for some people, communities or individuals.
    *   *Social determinants of health*: The socio-economic causes of health inequalities.

Annotated further reading

Dahlgren, G. and Whitehead, W. (2006) *European Strategies for Tackling Social Inequity in Health: Levelling Up Part 2*. Available at: www.euro.who.int/en/health-topics/health-determinants/social-determinants/publications/2007/european-strategies-for-tackling-social-inequalities-in-health-2

This document is a public health strategy aimed at reducing health inequalities in Europe, published by the European regional office of the WHO. Reading this document will enable you to see how public health initiatives are driven forward on an international scale. You could correlate the key points with your local trust's policy to see how they align, then discuss your findings with your supervisor or line manager.

Friel, S., Marmot, M., Bell, R., Houweling, T. and Taylor, S. (2008) *WHO Commission on Social Determinants of Health: Closing the Gap in a Generation*. Available at: www.who.int/social_determinants/thecommission/finalreport/en/

The WHO invested in collating evidence of how social factors influence health and health inequalities around the world into one document. The report is extensive and provides valuable details about many determinants of health. However, there is an executive summary that you can read if you need an overview rather than an in-depth discussion.

Public Health England (PHE) (2014) *Immunisations Against Infectious Disease: The Green Book*. Available at: www.gov.uk/government/collections/immunisation-against-infectious-disease-the-green-book#the-green-book

This is a weblink to *The Green Book*, a list of all licensed immunisations and vaccines in the UK. It is an important document for you to read and refer to if you are involved in administering any vaccinations. You will most likely be working in a community environment, such as a GP surgery, if you are going to administer vaccinations.

Williams, E., Buck, D. and Babalola, G. (2020) *What Are Health Inequalities?* Available at: www.kingsfund.org.uk/publications/what-are-health-inequalities

This is another very useful web page from the King's Fund about health inequalities. The information here is presented very clearly in a variety of diagrams and graphics accompanied by succinct descriptions. The information here also links with the social determinants of health, identified as 'wider determinants of health'. This is essential reading to understand health inequalities.

Useful websites

Genomics Education Programme: www.genomicseducation.hee.nhs.uk/education/

The material on this website is excellent and comprehensive, as well as being written to accommodate people with varying levels of knowledge about genomics. The majority of the online learning material is freely available, and you can download a certificate of completion to add to your CPD portfolio. With this in mind, you could set yourself an appraisal objective to complete one of HEE's online genomics courses. Remember to be able to discuss why you would like to learn more about genomics with your supervisor or line manager.

Genomics England: www.genomicsengland.co.uk

This website is an excellent resource of information about genomics in England. You can read more about the 100,000 Genomes Project, as well as the latest research and educational material. Genomics will play an important part in the future of healthcare, so investing time to understand genomics will be greatly beneficial. For more information about the future of health and social care, as well as the role you could play as a nursing associate, see Chapter 8.

Health Education England Training and Educational Resources: www.hee.nhs.uk/our-work/population-health/training-educational-resources

This web page is a repository of many very useful resources to help you enhance your public health practice. HEE has collated packs of information about a variety of public health topics that you can use to improve your knowledge and apply to your practice. The content is centred on protecting good health and reducing health inequalities by training healthcare professionals.

Public Health England: www.gov.uk/government/organisations/public-health-england

Visit this website for information about what PHE does, as well as how its work affects the national population and local communities. Use this website as a valid and reliable source of information about public health.

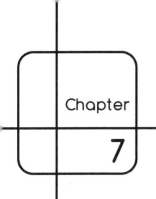

Chapter

7

Health promotion and practice education

(Continued)

4.7   support, supervise and act as a role model to nursing associate students, health care support workers and those new to care roles, review the quality of the care they provide, promoting reflection and providing constructive feedback

4.8   contribute to team reflection activities, to promote improvements in practice and services

Platform 6: Contributing to integrated care

At the point of registration, the nursing associate will be able to:

6.4   understand the principles and processes involved in supporting people and families with a range of care needs to maintain optimal independence and avoid unnecessary interventions and disruptions to their lives

Chapter aims

After reading this chapter, you will be able to:

- define health promotion and how it is related to public health;
- describe how health promotion initiatives can improve the health and wellbeing of patients and their family, friends and carers;
- develop methods to critically analyse health promotion initiatives;
- identify when to use the principles of practice education as a nursing associate;
- explain how practice education is within your scope of practice as a nursing associate.

Introduction

Chapter 6 was about public health and health inequalities for nursing associates. This chapter goes hand in hand with that chapter, as health promotion and practice education are parts of practice that contribute to public health and reduce health inequalities. During this chapter, we will explore how this can be achieved. The key themes we will discuss are how health promotion can improve the health and wellbeing of patients and their family, friends and carers. The themes will build on the principles of public health you learned about in Chapter 6 (i.e. promoting and protecting good health). Your ability to think critically will be developed during this chapter in relation to health promotion initiatives that contribute to person-centred care. To be able to include health promotion in your practice, you need to be able to apply the principles of practice education, and hence practice education is also included in this chapter. Teaching others can be a daunting experience, but this chapter includes fundamental principles of practice education to guide your practice. Remember that you already have many of the skills needed to be effective at practice education (e.g. communication, active listening, empathy), so remember to include these skills when working through the case studies in this chapter. Before reading the first section, consider the quotation below from the NMC *Standards of Proficiency for Nursing Associates*, which summarises your valuable contribution to promoting and protecting good health as a nursing associate:

Nursing associates play a role in supporting people to improve and maintain their mental, physical, behavioural health and wellbeing. They are actively involved in the prevention of and protection against disease and ill health, and engage in public health, community development, and in the reduction of health inequalities.

(NMC, 2018a, p7)

Health promotion and public health

Health promotion can be described as an action of public health. In other words, public health is focused on protecting and promoting good health, which is relative to each individual. Hence, health promotion is about implementing initiatives that enable and encourage a person to autonomously achieve their perception of good physical and psychological health (Edelman and Kudzma, 2018). Remember that each individual has unique interpretations of what is important for good health (e.g. physicality, psychology, spirituality, socio-economy), so you need to conduct a person-centred assessment to define the health that a patient is aiming to achieve.

There are many aims and principles of health promotion, and the next box summarises some key points for you to read. Overall, your practice should include the protection, prevention and promotion of health – these concepts implemented together can be described as health promotion. The WHO periodically organises an international conference on health promotion, the first being in 1986 in Ottawa, Canada. The conference reports are freely available for you to read; you will find a weblink to these in the useful websites section at the end of the chapter.

The health behaviours of patients are important for you to understand to enable you to provide person-centred health promotion. Health behaviours are the actions and activities of patients that positively or negatively impact health and morbidity (Short and Mollborn, 2015). Health behaviours are affected by patients' activities of daily living (ADLs) and their social determinants of health (Dahlgren and Whitehead, 2006; Roper et al., 2000). For more information on these two concepts, see Chapters 4 and 6, respectively. Health promotion involves supporting and enabling patients to autonomously maintain beneficial health behaviours and change negative health behaviours to achieve their health goals. This explanation is an example of how health promotion is closely linked with public health, and hence your actions as a nursing associate are imperative to effective health promotion.

The actions of health promotion, like all care interventions, should be person-centred. Think back to the five steps of the nursing process: assessment, patient goals, planning, implementation and evaluation (Howatson-Jones et al., 2015). The nursing process was discussed in depth in Chapter 2, and it was highlighted that these five steps can guide your practice in any circumstance of your practice. The context of Chapter 2 was acute and long-term care, but the nursing process is still relevant to health promotion.

First, you need to conduct a person-centred assessment of the patient's health behaviours. This does not involve seeking and pointing out all the negatives; highlighting positive health behaviours is more important because positive reinforcement is encouraging. Next establish the patient's good health goal. Ask them what their ideal description of 'good health' is, remembering to ensure that the goal is SMART (for more information, see Chapter 2). Once you know the patient's good health goal, you can plan what health promotion initiatives or education are needed to support the patient in achieving their goal. The implementation stage requires the patient to be autonomous, so make sure you have provided as much information as needed to empower the patient. Lastly, you can evaluate the health promotion initiatives that were implemented to establish why they were successful or not. Remember that the nursing process is cyclical, so you may need to establish a progressive number of small SMART goals that the patient can work towards in order to achieve their interpretation of good health. This may require multiple cycles of the nursing process, and an evaluation between each SMART goal will establish what does and does not work for the patient when trying to improve their health.

Understanding the theory: guiding principles of health promotion

There are a vast number of actions that you can implement to contribute to promoting good health and health behaviours of patients and their family, friends and carers. Similar to public health, health promotion is a broad subject with many different methods and models. Five principles of health promotion have been included here to give you some guidance on how to ensure that your practice promotes the health of the patients you are caring for, based on the Ottawa Charter for Health Promotion (WHO, 1986; see also Hubley and Copeman, 2013).

1. *Public health policy.* Make sure you read and understand international, national, regional and local health promotion policy. The local policy of the trust you work for will inform your day-to-day practice, whereas international, national and regional health promotion policy will provide you with context, and thus your understanding of health promotion will be more comprehensive. Also read other sources of health promotion literature and remember to discuss your findings with your supervisor or line manager to consolidate what you have learned.

2. *Establish inclusive environments.* Similar to providing care to patients, the environment must be welcoming, supportive and relaxed. Creating this atmosphere is important for implementing health promotion initiatives because patients need to feel comfortable to reflect on their own health behaviours. If patients feel antagonised, stressed or upset, they are less likely to have an open mind when reflecting on their health behaviours, and thus are less likely to feel motivated to make positive lifestyle choices. For more details on creating a rapport with patients, see Chapter 2.

3. *Encourage autonomy.* One of the defining principles of person-centred care is to provide as much empowerment to patients as is possible. As we have discussed before, one of the components of informed consent is adequate information. In relation to health promotion, empowerment and adequate information are combined together to encourage autonomy. In context, patients who have been educated about their health behaviours and the benefits of positive lifestyle choices are more informed, and hence are more likely to positively change their lifestyle, promoting and pro- tecting their good health.

4. *Strengthen family and community support.* Promoting health is only halfway to the desired outcome. To achieve promoted health, patients need to make positive lifestyle choices, which may mean

making substantial changes to their ADLs. Giving up smoking after a number of years, for example, is an extraordinarily difficult task. However, patients are often able to achieve their health promotion goals with the support of their family, friends and carers. Furthermore, we know from Chapter 6 that the social determinants of health affect our behaviour, so community support of health promotion is equally important. This could mean highlighting to a patient the accessible health promotion services that are in their community, such as a smoking cessation group. The more positive reinforcement the patient has about health promotion, the more likely they are to change their health behaviours.

5. *Health services direction.* The fourth principle highlights the importance of community services, but in addition to this patients should be informed about other health services available to them. Remember that health is both physical and psychological. Remember to discuss this with patients where appropriate to do so, particularly the benefits of making positive lifestyle choices for physical and mental health. A 30-minute jog or run, for example, is a positive lifestyle choice with physical and mental health benefits – and is free of charge. A family walk for 30 minutes has benefits too, which could include strengthening family relationships, as well as physical and mental health.

Remember that there is much more literature about health promotion, so do not limit your knowledge to these examples. Go to the annotated further reading section at the end of the chapter for some more sources of information on health promotion. Lastly, consider the inclusion of learning more about how you can promote health as a nursing associate, as part of your self-directed CPD.

The previous box provided you with some guiding principles of health promotion. The explanations of how they are relevant to your scope of practice as a nursing associate are examples of how these theoretical principles can be applied in practice. Remember that there is no singular way to conduct your practice, as every patient – and every situation you are in – is unique. The health promotion principles noted in the box are included to highlight how you can contribute to the health promotion of the patient you are caring for.

Person-centred health promotion

So far in this chapter, we have discussed some of the basic principles of health promotion. The nursing process is applicable to health promotion and can aid you in providing person-centred care. However, there is more you can do to ensure that your practice is person-centred. In this section, there are some examples of practical ways you can introduce health promotion, but first consider when it is appropriate to begin discussing a patient's health behaviours, and more importantly when it is not.

In the previous box, we already identified that the environment you conduct your care in must be inclusive, informal and relaxed enough for the patient to discuss the very personal topic of their health behaviours. What constitutes a relaxed environment can only be determined by the patient. If you work in the community, in the patient's home, this is usually an environment in which the patient feels most comfortable, although there are exceptions to this (e.g. if the patient's home is unsafe, physically or emotionally). Therefore, if you are caring for a patient in their home, this may be an opportune moment to discuss health promotion. However, if the patient is distressed, in pain or acutely unwell, it is evident that health promotion is not their first priority, and these circumstances are not an ideal opportunity to discuss health behaviours. Once again, there is no rulebook to instruct you when or when not to conduct health promotion. Basing your clinical intuition on the guiding principles discussed so far will help you.

Making every contact count (also referred to as MECC), written collaboratively by PHE and HEE, is another framework that can guide your practice in health promotion (PHE, 2018b). There are a series of guiding documents, and the implementation guide is of particular use for you as a nursing associate. The implementation guide is primarily for organisational leaders who intend to integrate MECC into their health system, but the eight steps within it can be used to inform your practice:

1. Read organisational policy and health promotion strategy.
2. Note direction of policy implementation from senior leaders.
3. Assess and plan how to conduct health promotion.
4. Identify resources you may need (for some examples, see Table 7.1).
5. Consider the most appropriate environment and timing for health promotion.
6. Implement health promotion practice.
7. Continuing professional development (CPD) – health promotion training.
8. Evaluate health promotion process.

PHE has also published an evaluation guide for MECC. The MECC evaluation guide is a clear, systematic process that can support you in evaluating your application of MECC, which links with the evaluation stages of the nursing process (Howatson-Jones et al., 2015; PHE, 2020). You can supplement your learning about MECC by going to the NICE website, which contains advice about developing a MECC health promotion approach for your practice; a weblink has been provided in the useful websites section at the end of the chapter.

Thinking back to the beginning of this chapter, health promotion was defined as promoting health from a holistic perspective (i.e. physical and psychological health). Often both types of health are interconnected, so your practice should reflect this. In other words, when you are practising health promotion, you should simultaneously implement physical and psychological health promotion initiatives. But how do you promote good mental health? The guiding principles referred to so far can be applied to mental health, but there are bespoke mental health promotion guiding principles. According to Barry (2019), mental health promotion should:

*   be inclusive of everyone in the MDT;
*   enhance protection methods of good mental health;
*   create supportive environments for good mental health;
*   provide access to mental health resources, services and networks (e.g. family and friends).

Reflecting on your practice to self-assess your adherence to these principles provides you with an opportunity to evaluate the effectiveness of your mental health promotion practice. For example, many people find listening to music comforting and a relief from stress or anxiety. This may be something you do after a long day at work. Have you ever considered what genre of music you listen to when you feel a certain way? When upset, some people listen to upbeat music to lift their mood, whereas others prefer to listen to sombre music to help them process their emotions. Neither option is right or wrong; what matters is enabling personal choice. Furthermore, involving family or friends in supporting patients who are having a period of mental health difficulties can strengthen the supportive environment the patient is in. Some examples of mental health promotion initiatives are provided in Table 7.1.

We have looked at many principles of health promotion so far in this chapter, but are there any for paediatric health promotion? In Chapter 6, it was highlighted that public health for children is very important because it provides an opportunity for preventive health behaviours to be adopted early on in a person's life. The earlier that positive health behaviours are adopted, the longevity of a healthy fulfilling life is increased. The WHO, with UNESCO, has written a concept note for developing a global standard for health promotion in schools, which is directly relevant for your practice as a nursing associate (WHO, 2018). In essence, the standard will aim to make every school an environment for health promotion. The concept note is useful to read because it describes the current climate of health promotion in schools and identifies potential challenges. You can use the principles outlined in this chapter so far to mitigate these challenges and promote health in schools that you may work in.

The wide variety of guiding principles outlined in this chapter so far can support you in ensuring that you are able to provide health promotion advice to patients and their family, friends and carers. Table 7.1 provides you with some practical examples of health promotion initiatives that you may choose to implement in your practice. Remember that there may be others available within your local area or online, so do some reading beforehand and discuss any new initiatives you would like to introduce to your practice with your supervisor or line manager.

Table 7.1   Health promotion initiative examples

Health promotion opportunity	Health promotion initiative and resource
Balanced diet	British Heart Foundation, *Eat Better* (BHF, 2019):
	www.bhf.org.uk/informationsupport/publications/healthy-eating-and-drinking/eat-better
Exercise	NHS, *10-Minute Workouts* (NHS, 2018c):
	www.nhs.uk/live-well/exercise/10-minute-workouts/
Mental health	Mind, *Mindfulness* (Mind, 2018):
	www.mind.org.uk/information-support/drugs-and-treatments/mindfulness/about-mindfulness/
Smoking	Royal College of Nursing, *Smoking Cessation* (RCN, 2020b):
	www.rcn.org.uk/clinical-topics/public-health/smoking-cessation

Table 7.1 provides you with some examples of initiatives that are available for you to use in clinical practice. As noted beforehand, new health promotion initiatives are periodically published, some of which may be more relevant to the patients you are caring for. Make sure that you thoroughly investigate the most appropriate health promotion initiative to use in your practice before implementing it, as well as checking with your supervisor or line manager for their advice. Most of all, remember to involve and include the patient's family, friends and carers with health promotion (if this is the patient's choice), because they can make valuable contributions in supporting the patient to make positive lifestyle choices and improve their health behaviours. Activity 7.1 provides you with an opportunity to apply your learning to a case study.

Activity 7.1   Critical thinking

You are working in a primary school with two children currently in your care, Hannah and Yūsuf. Hannah is diabetic and is feeling unwell because she did not eat her lunch. Yūsuf has autism and is currently crying because there are too many loud noises in the room. You are with the teaching assistant, Mrs Zarah, and the teacher, Mr Simon, has gone to get a first aid kit that contains the medicine to treat Hannah's hypoglycaemia. In this situation, what should you do?

Remember that you need to be able to prioritise and manage your workload as a nursing associate, which means being able to use resources effectively and recognising when it is safe to delegate care provision to your colleagues. Use your critical thinking skills to evaluate the safest course of action for Hannah and Yūsuf.

An outline answer is provided at the end of the chapter.

Activity 7.1 encourages you to think about the combination of acute and long-term care while managing more than one patient and working with others. In addition to supporting patients with health promotion, you need to remember to look after your own health. This is covered in depth in Chapter 8, but read the next section for information relating to your own health promotion.

Nursing associate health and wellbeing

We have discussed health promotion of patients and their family, friends and carers in depth in this chapter so far. But what about your own health and wellbeing as a nursing associate? The *Standards of Proficiency for Nursing Associates* states that you must recognise how your own fitness, health and wellbeing affect your practice (NMC, 2018a). In other words, as registered practitioners, we need to promote our own health as well as the health of our patients. This will not only enable us to practise, but also to achieve a long, healthy and fulfilling life. While many practitioners know and understand the components of healthy living, it can sometimes be a challenge to adopt positive health behaviours. After working a busy 11-hour shift, for example, it is likely that you will be dehydrated if you have not drunk enough water during your shift, and you may feel too tired to cook a healthy meal when you arrive home. Eating fast food is a tempting alternative – while choosing this option can be an occasional treat, repetitively eating fast food is damaging to your health. It is likely that you already know this, so what can you do to maintain positive health behaviours? Preparing meals on a day off is one technique that some practitioners adopt to manage this challenge, but there are many alternatives. For more suggestions on good health behaviours for nursing associates, see Chapter 8.

Similar to patients, you need to ensure that you look after your mental health. A career as a nursing associate, or any health or social care professional, includes stressful days. Just as you provide person-centred health promotion to patients, take time to find what strategies work to promote your own positive mental health. Reflection will play an important part in processing stressful days. Reflection can help you to identify learning points, including how to maintain and improve good practice, but can also help you to recognise coping mechanisms for any future stressful days. For more examples of how to promote your mental health as a nursing associate, see Chapter 8.

As a registered nursing associate, you may need to lead a small team of healthcare support workers, or supervise an apprentice nursing associate or student. With this in mind, how do you support your colleagues and act as a role model for not only evidence-based, person-centred care, but also positive health behaviours? Encouraging others to have positive health behaviours will strengthen your working relationships, such as ensuring that the people you are supervising have time for a break when it is appropriate to do so. Even during busy days, breaks are paramount to reduce the risk of practitioners becoming overtired and making errors, which may cause harm to patients. However, be mindful of your own health behaviours. For example, are you able to offer smoking cessation advice to patients or colleagues if you are a smoker yourself? This is an interesting point of debate. Some people may think that you are unable to give smoking cessation advice when you are a smoker because you are a bad role model. Consider the alternative, which is if you are a smoker who is also trying to stop smoking – you understand exactly what it feels like. This experience may make you more empathetic to patients and colleagues who are progressing towards giving up smoking. An important point to remember here is honesty. Sharing your true experience, within professional boundaries, with patients and colleagues could be a way of building trust and a rapport.

When supervising others, remember that you are in a privileged position to support them in developing their practice. In relation to health promotion, you may have asked a final year apprentice nursing associate to advise a patient on how they can eat more healthily while being supervised by you. As a responsible supervisor, you will have checked that the apprentice nursing associate is confident and competent enough to provide this advice. Following this episode of care, there is an opportunity for you to provide some constructive feedback and facilitate reflection. This does not mean that you reflect for the apprentice nursing associate, but you encourage them to identify what they did well and how they could improve. Remember that constructive feedback is never negative; it always includes positives and identifies areas for improvement. Reflection and constructive feedback about health promotion can be for an individual, or you could facilitate a team discussion within the area you work to contribute to service improvement.

Practice education and health promotion

Practice education usually refers to the education of health and social care practitioners. It refers to learning in a formal classroom setting or within clinical practice. The topic of practice education is very large, considering that the education of practitioners involves academic study and training for professional registration. For example, as a nursing associate, you are working towards a foundation degree in science and your NMC registration. Practice education, however, also includes patient education, and requires you to be involved in the teaching of patients and their family and friends. In other words, during your nursing associate education, you will learn how to teach patients and their family, friends and carers, as well as your colleagues. This section of the chapter will provide you with some guiding principles of practice education in relation to health promotion.

Practice education is directly relevant to health promotion because when patients understand the impact of their health behaviours, they are more likely to make positive lifestyle choices (Sharma, 2016). It is likely that you already have some experience in practice education. You may have taught a patient how to change their **stoma** bag for the first time or taught another patient about their new diagnosis of **Raynaud's syndrome**. This is evidence of how practice education is an integral part of your role as a nursing associate.

Regardless of whether you have some experience of practice education or none at all, understanding the principles of practice education can enhance your abilities. Some suggestions for each stage of educating a patient and their family, friends and carers, or a colleague, are listed below:

1. *Aim.* Before teaching someone, you need to identify an aim for the session (i.e. the end product of the session). Limiting the number of aims ensures that your teaching session does not become overly complex – one aim is usually enough in clinical practice. Trying to include too many aims decreases the chance of the person you are teaching remembering what you have said.

2. *Objectives.* The objectives are the small, progressive steps that you and the learner need to achieve in order to achieve the aim. Similar to the aim, keep things simple and manageable. Be mindful of the amount of time you have and the resources available – both time and resources can be limited in a high-pressured clinical environment. Make sure that you share the aim and objectives with the patient or your colleague so that they know what to expect and can make some requests about the session. For example, they may want to have things written down, in which case you know to give them a handout.

3. *Informal pretest against learning outcome.* Most people become anxious when a test is introduced; however, this stage is not a formal test like you have at university. You are simply establishing what the person already knows. By doing so, you will not need to repeat certain points.

4. *Learning and teaching activities.* This stage is when you actively teach the person. There are many parallels between practice education and clinical practice, such as ensuring that you are using effective communication and that you have a person-centred approach. Depending on how much time you have, consider including a variety of activities when teaching, rather than limiting yourself to a verbal description (e.g. using leaflets as a visual aid).

5. *Post-test against learning outcomes.* The post-test is similarly informal. At this stage, you are checking that the person has achieved each learning outcome you agreed at the beginning, achieved the aim, and learned sufficient information or a new skill.

6. *Evaluation.* Lastly, seek feedback from the person you have taught. Their comments of what they enjoyed or thought could have gone better will only improve your practice. Use their evaluation to reflect on this experience as this will consolidate what you have learned about practice education.

(Williams and Rutter, 2019)

Remember that each situation and patient you care for are different, so always ensure that you have a person-centred approach to practice education and health promotion. Complete Activity 7.2 to identify how you could apply each stage of practice education in context.

Activity 7.2   Critical thinking

You are a nursing associate working in a cardiology outpatient clinic. The patient you are caring for, Alex, has just been diagnosed with hypertension. The cardiologist has briefly explained what the long-term condition is, but when escorting the patient out he tells you that he did not understand what the doctor told him and was too embarrassed to ask the doctor to repeat it. He asks you to clarify what the doctor said. Alex's hypertension is mild and can be controlled through diet and exercise.

What would you say to Alex? Remember to use your critical thinking skills to assess what is the most appropriate course of action to support Alex.

An outline answer is provided at the end of the chapter.

Chapter summary

This chapter is closely related to Chapter 6 on public health. To provide public health, you need to be able to promote and protect people's health. This chapter provides you with guidance and suggestions on how to do this. Remember to choose an appropriate time and location to discuss with patients how they can promote their own health. Involving their family, friends and carers is important so that they can provide motivational support during periods of adjustment to a healthier lifestyle. However, health promotion is impossible to achieve without practice education. Practice education involves being able to use teaching skills to educate patients about their health and the potential benefits if they make more positive lifestyle choices. Similar to discussing health promotion initiatives, when educating patients, make sure that you have appropriate timing and a suitable location which is safe for both you and the patient.

Practice education also involves your colleagues within the MDT. You may have learned new skills or gained new knowledge from your CPD, and sharing this will contribute to their development, as well as consolidating your understanding. In both health promotion and practice education, you will need to use your critical thinking skills to ensure that you apply the most valid and reliable evidence to your practice.

Activities: Brief outline answers

Activity 7.1 Critical thinking (page 105)

Hannah and Yūsuf both require care, a mixture of acute and long-term needs. Hannah is hypoglycaemic and requires fast acting sugar, followed by complex carbohydrates to maintain her capillary blood glucose level within safe parameters. Yūsuf is clearly distressed by the situation and needs to be moved to a more calm, quiet environment. Out of the two children, Hannah is the most acutely unwell, but Yūsuf needs to be cared for too in another room. You know from the case study description that a first aid kit is being brought to you by Mr Simon. In the room is yourself and Mrs Zahra. As the experienced healthcare practitioner, it is safer for you to remain with Hannah because you are trained to care for patients who are unwell. Mrs Zahra may have some first aid training and will be skilled in communication with children. With this in mind, it is safe for you to ask Mrs Zahra to take Yūsuf into another room and give him some support. At this point, you have managed the acute situation, but is there an opportunity for any health promotion? Once Hannah has had her medicine and eaten something, you can begin to explain to her the importance of eating a balanced lunch to keep her healthy. Once Yūsuf is feeling more relaxed, you could suggest to him some strategies for managing anxiety, such as removing himself from the situation and practising mindfulness. Both of these examples are health promotion – Hannah's physical health and Yūsuf's mental health. In practice you will need to adapt your practice and communication to ensure that both children can understand the health advice you are providing. Lastly, remember you should include the children's family in health promotion. Consider if it is appropriate for you to share with the parents or guardians what health promotion technique work and those that do not for Hannah and Yūsuf. Discuss any alternative ways of managing this case study you can think of with your supervisor or line manager.

Activity 7.2 Critical thinking (page 108)

Alex has told you that he felt embarrassed to ask the doctor to repeat what was said during the consultation. Thinking back to the principles of health promotion, you need to ensure that the environment is inclusive and relaxed so that Alex feels comfortable enough to reflect on his health behaviours. You could take him into another consultation room, for example, so that his privacy and dignity are maintained. In the private space, identify the aim and objectives. The aim could be for Alex to understand hypertension, and the objectives may be to define the condition and describe what changes Alex needs to make (one aim and two objectives). Next is the pretest, so you could ask Alex if he knows anything about hypertension, also known as high blood pressure. He may say that he has heard of it but knows nothing about it. Now you know that you need to start from the basics, explaining to Alex that high blood pressure is when his heart is beating harder than expected for his age.

You could then explain the likely causes, which could be limited exercise, an unbalanced diet, smoking or drinking. Alex may tell you that he does not smoke and only drinks socially but recognises that he could do more exercise and eat healthy foods more often. You can now work together with Alex to determine when and how he could exercise and suggest ways to improve his diet – you could refer back to the resources mentioned earlier in this chapter. Once you have taught Alex these points, you can conduct the post-test by asking him if there is anything else that he would like to know, as well as if he thinks he achieved the aim and objectives that you set out at the beginning. If there is nothing more, ask him for his feedback on how this session was helpful, document clearly in his patient record, and reflect on this experience at a later time. Remember to discuss your reflections and what you learned from the experience with your supervisor or line manager.

Annotated further reading

Esterhuizen, P. (2019) *Reflective Practice in Nursing*, 4th edition. London: SAGE/Learning Matters.

This book is about reflective practice. Reflection is an important part of both health promotion and practice education. When teaching patients about an acute or long-term condition, or about a new skill, reflecting on the experience will help you to identify what you did well and how to improve for next time.

Evans, D., Coutsaftiki, D. and Fathers, C. (2017) *Health Promotion and Public Health for Nursing Students*, 3rd edition. London: SAGE.

This book is relevant to Chapters 6 and 7. Although written for nursing students, much of the content is also relevant to nursing associates. There is an emphasis on how to support people to make positive lifestyle choices, as well as important considerations for public health.

King's Fund (2019a) *Public Health: Our Position*. Available at: www.kingsfund.org.uk/projects/positions/public-health

This online article from the King's Fund links Chapters 6 and 7 together. Public health, practice education and health promotion are interconnected, as many public health concerns can be improved through health promotion and patient education. This article provides you with the context of public health at the time of publication. Reading it will enable you to have a wider understanding of public health, health promotion and patient education. Remember to check for updates on the King's Fund website to ensure that you are reading the most up-to-date material.

Useful websites

National Institute for Health and Care Excellence – Making Every Contact Count: https://stpsupport.nice.org.uk/mecc/index.html#article

This web page contains advice about how to develop your health promotion practice according to the MECC guidance. There are many links to other resources, so the information provided for you via this web page is extensive.

Public Health England – Making Every Contact Count Resources: www.makingevery contactcount.co.uk/national-resources/

Visit this web page for a variety of resources to inform your knowledge and guide your practice in MECC, a framework for health promotion. The guidance published here is transferable to any practice environment, and hence it is ideal for nursing associates who work in all four fields of nursing.

World Health Organization Global Health Promotion Conferences: www.who.int/ healthpromotion/conferences/en/

This weblink will take you to the list of all past conference reports that the WHO has conducted. Reading the reports will provide you with information on how health promotion has evolved over time, as well as the progress that has been made. More importantly, the most recent report provides advice for current health promotion practice.

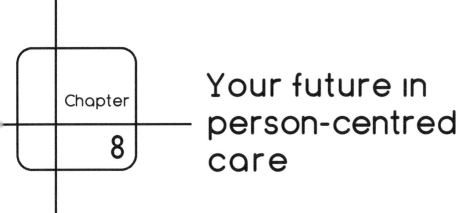

Your future in person-centred care

Chapter

8

(Continued)

Platform 5: Improving safety and quality of care

At the point of registration, the nursing associate will be able to:

5.6   understand and act in line with local and national organisational frameworks, legislation and regulations to report risks, and implement actions as instructed, following up and escalating as required

Chapter aims

After reading this chapter, you will be able to:

- define the nursing associate scope of practice and the interrelation with the MDT;
- recognise the literacy, numeracy, digital and technology skills needed to fulfil the role of a nursing associate;
- describe how team-working and leadership are important for person-centred care;
- have an awareness of the potential future developments in the health services and the valuable contribution that nursing associates can make to person-centred care.

Introduction

This book has provided you with pointers in the right direction to develop your person-centred approach to care. One of the privileges of working in health and social care is that there is always something new to learn or develop. The final chapter of this book focuses on your future as a nursing associate providing person-centred care. Reading this chapter will provide you with suggestions on how to continually enhance your person-centred practice while maintaining currency as the political, socio-economic landscapes shift. Healthcare services and systems will constantly evolve, and you need to ensure that your practice evolves too. One example is the increasing use of technology to support healthcare practitioners to provide person-centred care. This chapter also includes advice on effective time management, team-working and leadership, which will support you to become an ambassador for the nursing associate profession. The chapter will conclude with thoughts for the future. The NHS will be a completely different organisation by the end of the twenty-first century, and your person-centred practice as a nursing associate will help to shape it.

Nursing associate scope of practice

Throughout this book, there have been many reminders to ensure that you stay within your scope of practice. As the NHS and health services develop over time, it is important that you remain familiar with your scope of practice in order to ensure that your practice is safe – consider this as your 'safe zone' in providing person-centred care. The NMC *Standards of Proficiency for Nursing*

Associates are absolutely key to defining your scope of practice. You will have noticed that each chapter of this book has been mapped with these standards, so you can clearly see how the content is relevant to your practice (NMC, 2018a). What can be potentially difficult to define is where the boundaries of your scope of practice are, and where those of other members of the MDT begin.

Knowing where the boundaries of your scope of practice are not only provides you with professional security; it equips you with the knowledge to explain to others what you can and cannot do for patients. This leads to the most important reason why you need to know your scope of practice: it keeps patients safe. Even in a highly functional healthcare team, people can be presumptious about what other members of the MDT have done or will do for patients. In these circumstances, there is a risk that important patient care will be overlooked because everyone has presumed that someone else has done it or will do it. Therefore, clear communication among the team mitigates the risk of care omissions. Knowing the scope of the MDT members' scopes of practice is helpful too. You do not need to know them in detail, but knowing where to look for them is important. Reading them can also help you to know what you can ask each member of the MDT to do for patients, which can help you feel confident in **delegation**. See the useful websites section at the end of the chapter for weblinks to the four health and social care governing body websites.

Confidently knowing how to interact with, support and motivate others in the MDT is important for promoting and providing safe person-centred care. These concepts summarise the principles of team-working, which are discussed later in this chapter. For now, consider why effective teamwork is needed for the provision of person-centred care. Each member of the MDT makes unique contributions to patient care; no one member can do everything for patients, and equally if one member of the MDT was removed their subject matter expertise would be lost. In this unlikely circumstance, the provision of holistic patient care would be incomplete. As nursing associates are generalist practitioners and a common thread throughout the MDT, you are able to interact with, support and motivate members of the MDT. In context, this may mean ensuring that communication between team members is efficient, or alternatively advocating patients' choices during shift handovers. These are examples of how you can interact with and support members of the MDT. Supplementing these actions with **positive reinforcement** is an example of how to motivate members of the MDT. Positive reinforcement is a type of feedback that is used to recognise achievements or exemplary practice, and the impact is motivation for the recipient (Prestia, 2017). Positive reinforcement must be a genuine, honest acknowledgement of excellent person-centred practice. Motivating others' person-centred practice in the MDT is also a method to promote person-centred practice. This is especially important when you are using delegation.

Delegation is the act of a registered practitioner, such as a nursing associate, asking a colleague to carry out a care intervention or activity (RCNI, 2017). It is important to understand that delegating something to a colleague because you do not want to do it is extremely poor practice and a sign of weak **leadership**. You should only delegate if it provides you with the opportunity to carry out another high-priority care intervention or activity that you would not be able to do otherwise. However, you must make sure that the person you are delegating to meets the following criteria:

- is confident and competent to complete what has been delegated to them;
- has received training and passed a competency assessment of the care intervention or activity delegated to them;
- the delegated activity is within their scope of practice;
- the desired outcome of the delegated activity and instructions to achieve the outcome have been clearly explained, and an opportunity for clarifying questions has been provided;
- appropriate supervision is provided;
- documentation of the delegated activity is completed.

(RCNI, 2017)

Even though you have delegated a care intervention or activity to a colleague who meets the above criteria, you are still **accountable** for the intervention or activity. Your colleague is **responsible** for the care intervention or activity if they have provided their consent (to reiterate the differences between accountability and responsibility, see the definitions in the glossary). Activity 8.1 gives an example of poor delegation and an appropriate response.

Activity 8.1 Critical thinking and reflection

The Royal College of Nursing Institute (RCNI) produced an audio recording as a case study of a healthcare assistant being delegated a task outside their scope of practice. The healthcare assistant is put under pressure to carry out the care intervention, but confidently and professionally declines. They offer alternative support for the nurse who is delegating the care intervention. Listen to the audio recording via the weblink below (there is also a link to a downloadable transcript):

- RCNI audio recording: **https://soundcloud.com/user-680565483/delegation**
- Downloadable transcript (available at the bottom of this web page): **https://rcni.com/ hosted-content/rcn/first-steps/delegation**

After listening to the audio recording, reflect on the conversation and use your critical thinking skills to consider how the healthcare assistant was politely assertive and remained professional. Critically analyse how the registered nurse could have acted differently. Discuss your reflections with your supervisor or line manager. Lastly, remember to always adhere to the principles of delegation to ensure that you and your colleagues and patients are kept safe.

An outline answer is available at the end of the chapter, but remember that your own reflection will be individual.

The healthcare assistant in the audio recording of Activity 8.1 is an example of how to be an effective team member. As a registered nursing associate, Activity 8.1 is an example of how not to delegate, and completing the critical reflection will help you to consolidate your learning. In practice, if you have delegated a care intervention or activity to someone, you need to ensure that you provide supervision and support to promote the safety of your colleague and the patient. In other words, you need to be able to monitor and review the quality of care that you you provide, as well as the quality of care of others who you have delegated to.

Being able to monitor and review the quality of the care you provide, as well as that of others who have carried out care interventions or activities on your behalf, is another patient safety mechanism. It can also contribute to the development of both your own practice and that of your colleagues. Practice development may remind you of reflection, which is a valid and reliable method of monitoring and reviewing the quality of care. Usually, reflection takes place after an episode of care, to reflect back on your strengths and areas for development. However, reflection can be used as a continuing process during a care intervention or activity (Esterhuizen, 2019). Using a theoretical model as a guide for your active reflection can help you to critique your own practice as you are providing it. Practising this regularly will be beneficial for you, because to revalidate as a nursing associate with the NMC you need to record reflections in your portfolio that will be submitted for review. Supporting colleagues to actively reflect encourages everyone to autonomously monitor the quality of care, whereas facilitating a post-activity reflection can be a valuable learning exercise for the colleague you have delegated something to.

Chapter 7 was about health promotion, during which you were reminded to be mindful of your own health and wellbeing. Feeling physically and psychologically healthy enables you to provide compassionate person-centred care for patients. Think back to Chapter 1 and the 'Understanding the theory' box about Betari's box (Mind Tools, 2019a). This model represents how your attitudes and behaviours affect other people's attitudes and behaviours – colleagues and patients, as well as their family, friends and carers. To highlight another key point related to self-care, stress is important for you to manage. In health and social care, stress is inevitable. A small amount of stress is healthy as it motivates us to provide the best quality person-centred care. However, too much stress can lead to burnout and friction within a team. With this in mind, make sure to have regular reflections and discuss your thoughts and feelings with a trusted colleague, particularly when it has been a stressful day. Similarly, use your active listening skills for colleagues who are feeling stressed. These are positive actions that motivate the team you are working in, ultimately benefiting person-centred care for patients. Although stress is inevitable, it is manageable with the appropriate support. Effective time management can also make you feel in control of your own practice.

Many people defer to saying that there is no time to complete an intervention or care activity when under pressure. However, there is no such thing as having 'no time' (time is a constant law of physics, and there is an endless amount of time), but there is effective time management. Imagine for a moment that you were given £86,400 tomorrow morning. How would you spend it? Now imagine that you were given another £86,400 every morning for the rest of your life, but you cannot use any of the money you were given the day before. Each day you have to spend all of the £86,400 or you will lose the unspent amount. While having this amount of money each morning is a pleasurable thought, you are already being given 86,400 of another currency every day each time the clock resets. There are 86,400 seconds in every day (24 hours), and it is true that if you do not spend the 86,400 seconds wisely, you will lose the wasted seconds completely. Within the 24 hours of a day, clearly you need to spend a sufficient amount of time asleep, eating and drinking, and time with family and friends. The time you spend at work is also calculable in seconds, so you could work out how many seconds you spend at work during a shift. Therefore, the previous point about there being no such thing as having 'no time' is proven true. The important question for you as a nursing associate is: How do you choose to spend your time at work?

Effective time management for a nursing associate is about wisely using the amount of time available to provide evidence-based, person-centred care, as well as minimising any inefficiencies. As in all clinical environments, each situation and patient are different. How long it takes you to bathe one patient will be completely different to another patient who has a dermatological condition such as **psoriasis** or a **burn** injury. With this in mind, the following box contains some general principles of time management that you can use to promote the effective use of time in your and others' practice.

Understanding the theory: time management

Effective time management is situational and changes with each environment you work in, the patients you are caring for, and the time of day. The following principles of time management will guide your practice and support you in effectively using the time available to you during your shift:

(Continued)

(Continued)

1. *Arrive in plenty of time for your shift.* This provides you with an opportunity to read the handover sheets and plan your working day.

2. *Write notes.* Writing notes on your handover sheet or scrap paper enables you to physically see the care interventions and activities that you need to achieve, as well as mitigating the risk of something being forgotten. Remember to dispose of your notes in the confidential waste.

3. *Estimate how long each care intervention or activity will take.* On your notes, write down how long each care intervention or activity will approximately take. The timings will inform your plan for the day and ensure that you have a balanced workload for the time available.

4. *Prioritise.* Prioritise your workload from the perspective of patients, not how long a care intervention or activity will take. This will ensure that your provision of person-centred care is maintained.

5. *Minimise spontaneity.* Do not take on additional workload that is not a priority, even if it is easy to complete. Maintain your focus on the priority list you have written to avoid interruptions to patient care, unless there is an emergency that you can help to manage.

6. *Effective teamwork.* Always work in collaboration with your colleagues. If the MDT worked in silos (independently), progress would be slow and the quality of patient care would decrease. Refer to Activity 8.1 and the principles of delegation for guidance on how to politely remain focused on your workload when needed but offer support to your colleagues when you are able to.

7. *Take refreshment breaks.* Nursing and healthcare professionals are notoriously bad at having refreshment breaks. However, without these you become tired and the quality of your person-centred care is at risk. Make sure that you work with your colleagues in a shift to ensure that everyone has an opportunity for a refreshment break, which will help to maintain a positive work environment for staff and patients.

8. *Have flexibility and an open mind.* Sometimes a shift may become extremely busy, and the plan you made at the beginning of the day may not work out or a colleague may ask you to help with something important. It is important to remember that your plan is not set in stone – it is flexible. This is needed to ensure that all patients in the healthcare service you are in receive the person-centred care which they deserve.

9. *Avoid self-criticism.* If your plan does change or you have not completed everything on your list, do not be overly critical of yourself. Our work environment can be unpredictable and is always dynamic. Other priorities may have arisen during your shift that meant you were not able to achieve what you initially set out to do. This is fine. Remember that the ultimate priority for everyone in the MDT is to provide person-centred care. If this has been achieved, then you have had a successful day.

10. *Listen to patients.* The patients you are caring for are everyone's priority, and you can only provide person-centred care by actively listening to them. When writing your plan for the day or actively reflecting on your practice, ask the patients you are caring for what their priorities are to ensure that you are providing person-centred care (see the nursing process in Chapter 1).

(Woogara, 2012)

Apply these principles of time management to your practice to help you achieve effective time management, but remember that each situation is different, so you may need to adapt your strategy to provide person centred care. Discuss your potential strategies with your supervisor or line manager for advice on how to enhance your plans.

Effective time management has been proven to minimise stress and anxiety in clinical practice (Nayak, 2018). Therefore, it is in your interest to practise effective time management as a method to manage stress and anxiety. You can use the ten principles of effective time management from the previous box to guide your practice. You may also be able to advise colleagues you are supervising about time management as a tool to manage stress. Time management advice may be given when providing constructive feedback after a colleague has completed a care intervention or activity for you that you have delegated to them. With this in mind, providing constructive feedback is also important for you to be mindful of in your role as a nursing associate. Activity 8.2 provides you with an opportunity to reflect on your own experience of receiving feedback.

Activity 8.2   Reflection

It is likely that you will have had feedback from your supervisor, line manager or patients before. Using a reflection model, think back to a time when you received negative feedback. When someone provides negative feedback, they focus all of their attention on what – in their opinion – was wrong about what you did, avoid mentioning any of your strengths, and do not provide you with any advice on how to improve. If you have received negative feedback before, it is likely that you felt unmotivated and your confidence was damaged. While this is an unfortunate circumstance, reflecting on the experience can reiterate how you should not make the same errors – and never provide negative feedback.

Critically reflect on another time when you were enthused and motivated by feedback. The time when you felt motivated and enthused is likely to be because of the way the feedback was presented to you. Feedback should always be a positive experience for the recipient. This still includes discussing areas for improvement, but in a constructive way. When you give feedback to a colleague you have delegated a care intervention or activity to, or someone has asked you to give them feedback, you need to ensure that the feedback you give is both positive and constructive. It can be challenging to avoid being negative if someone has lots of room for improvement, but this is never an excuse for negative feedback (regardless of the experiences you have had in the past). Discuss your reflections on feedback with your supervisor or line manager. Consider asking about their reflections and experiences on receiving feedback.

As this activity is based on your own reflection, there is no outline answer provided at the end of the chapter.

The next box lists the principles of feedback that you can use to guide you on how to present feedback to colleagues. Providing feedback takes practice, particularly when concentrating to ensure that the feedback you are providing is constructive. Furthermore, providing constructive feedback to senior and/or experienced colleagues requires a lot of confidence. However, following the guidance in the next box will guide you.

Understanding the theory: constructive feedback

There are many tools that you can use when providing feedback to a colleague. You may be familiar with the model of starting feedback with a positive or strength, then suggesting an

(Continued)

(Continued)

area of development, and concluding with another positive or strength. This is an effective method because the emphasis of the feedback is the positives or strengths. People can still learn from identifying their strengths, as they may not have realised them. Highlighting negatives knocks people's confidence, but suggesting an area of development – and how to do this – is constructive and motivating, as well as promoting independent learning.

There are many alternative feedback tools that you may choose to use in practice. However, there are some guiding principles that you should adhere to, whichever feedback tool you choose to use:

1. *Feedback is an opportunity for development.* Professional development is beneficial for anyone in the MDT – most of all patients. Feedback is an informal, efficient method for professional development.

2. *Providing constructive feedback requires practice.* Presenting feedback can be challenging, particularly to a colleague who you consider a friend or to someone who is nervous or anxious. Therefore, practise giving feedback whenever it is appropriate for you to do so, and seek feedback on your feedback from your supervisor or line manager.

3. *Effective communication is essential.* Advanced communication skills are required to ensure that the feedback you provide is positive and constructive. Pay close attention to the recipient's body language and always provide feedback in a private space without an audience. Consider asking your supervisor or line manager to accompany you when giving feedback (with the recipient's informed consent) for additional support and contributions to the conversation.

4. *Focus on person-centred care and patient safety.* Feedback should be related back to person-centred care and patient safety. An activity you have delegated to a colleague may not directly involve patient care, but highlighting the indirect impact for patients is important for colleagues to understand why the activity needed completing, as well as how they supported you to provide person-centred care to another patient.

5. *Always be positive and constructive.* There is never an excuse for you to give negative feedback, even if you have received negative feedback yourself in the past. Receiving negative feedback can be difficult to process, so if this has happened to you, make sure that you discuss your reflection on this experience with a senior trusted colleague or your supervisor or line manager. Similarly, invest time in actively listening to someone who has received negative feedback and support them to recognise their positives and strengths.

6. *Promote reflection.* Encourage people to reflect on their practice when you have given your feedback. Reflection is an important skill in clinical practice, and it can be used to recognise the strengths and areas for development of person-centred care.

7. *Be honest and open to feedback.* Seek feedback on your own practice. This requires a significant amount of self-confidence, but remember that every time you receive feedback, it is a contribution to your professional development. Feedback from others can also help you to recognise something you may not have noticed yourself, as well as enriching your learning from reflection.

(Altmiller et al., 2018)

Providing positive and constructive feedback is another method to motivate colleagues, earn respect and develop your professional relationships with the MDT. Ultimately, you represent the profession of nursing associates, and positive, constructive feedback demonstrates your leadership and teamworking abilities.

The previous box provided you with some principles of effective feedback. You can use them in practice to guide you in providing feedback, but remember that each situation and person are different, so you may need to adapt the way you present positive and constructive feedback. Providing feedback to colleagues is part of effective teamwork and leadership. This is particularly important when you are supervising others or supporting a colleague in the MDT with a different professional background to your own. Therefore, understanding what constitutes effective team-working and leadership is paramount to your role as a nursing associate.

Team-working and leadership

As previously mentioned, teamwork within the MDT is integral to providing person-centred care. It is likely that you already have experience of team-working because the focus and motivation of the MDT is the patient. This is the difference between a group of people and a team – a group of people simply have a common interest or are together at the same time in the same place, whereas a team has a common goal that they are working towards achieving. Some teams are more effective than others. Common traits of an effective team are:

- effective communication;
- trust;
- rapport (professional working relationship);
- mutual respect and recognition of contributions;
- collaboration (working together);
- mitigating and managing conflict and disagreement.

(Souza et al., 2016)

Within a team, a leader is important to provide direction and facilitate everyone's contribution. Even if you are not leading a team, you still need to support your leader because the common goal is to provide person-centred care. Sometimes, however, you may need to use leadership skills too.

Many professionals not in a senior position believe that they are not leaders. However, every professional requires leadership skills in their roles. For nursing associates, you may be leading a small group of healthcare support workers, students or apprentices. In these circumstances, you will be using leadership skills. There are different models of leadership that are appropriate for different situations in clinical practice. Autocratic leadership is very direct and transactional. If you are using autocratic leadership, you will be instructing people what to do, without any debate. This style of leadership is very authoritarian and only appropriate in time-critical circumstances such as an emergency. Autocratic leadership is not appropriate in non-urgent situations, as it can be seen as controlling, overbearing or domineering, and team-working relationships can be damaged. A democratic leadership style is significantly more inclusive. Democratic leadership encourages team-workers to be included in the decision-making process, facilitated by the leader. It complements team-working and can lead to more effective decision-making because more than one person has contributed. The final leadership style mentioned here is transformational leadership. This is a style that focuses on leading people while simultaneously facilitating their professional development (Fischer, 2017). Transformational leadership is similar to democratic leadership, but also includes reflection and constructive feedback to promote the development of the people you are leading. For more material on leadership in healthcare practice, see the annotated further reading section at the end of the chapter.

When working within or leading a team, everyone must understand and have **concordance** with local policy, as well as national guidance and legislation, to ensure patient safety. Concordance with these documents is not simply a matter of complying with them. To have concordance is to have an understanding of what the framework, legislation or regulation is, how to adhere to them, and why this is important. Understanding these documents mitigates the risk of patients being harmed and protects healthcare professionals and team members. To achieve this understanding, you need to read the documents and clarify anything you are unsure of with your supervisor or line manager. By doing so, you will be demonstrating safe practice and awareness of the boundaries of your scope of practice and competence. If a colleague approaches you for clarification, make sure that you fully understand the framework, legislation or regulation before explaining it to them. If you are not sure, do not improvise. Simply state that you are unsure, but you can both go to your supervisor or line manager to find out together. This sets a very good example to your colleague and will also strengthen your knowledge. Activity 8.3 focuses on researching your local trust's policy on reporting risks and hazards.

Activity 8.3   Research

Reporting risks and hazards is another important contribution that you can make to the MDT as a nursing associate, demonstrating leadership in workplace and patient safety. Your health and safety mandatory training for your employer may have included how to report risks and hazards safely. Policies are periodically updated, so it is important to ensure that you have an up-to-date understanding and working knowledge of how to report risks and hazards in the workplace.

For this activity, take the time to read and understand your local trust's policy regarding reporting risks and hazards. Even if you have read it before, reread the policy and check for any updates. Doing so will ensure that your practice is up to date in relation to reporting risks and hazards. Remember that a hazard is a potential source or cause of harm, whereas a risk is the likelihood that a hazard will cause harm.

You could complete this activity as part of your CPD training or in preparation for your revalidation as a nursing associate with the NMC. Discuss your findings with your supervisor or line manager and ask for clarification on any uncertainties you have.

As this activity is based on your own reflection, there is no outline answer provided at the end of the chapter.

Completing Activity 8.3 enables you to update your knowledge and practice of reporting risks and hazards in the workplace, which promotes the safety of colleagues and patients. If you have reported a risk or hazard, your job is still not complete. When action has been taken to mitigate a risk or remove a hazard, or you have reported a risk or hazard, you need to check the outcome to ensure that the environment is safe and your documentation is accurate. Checking that the risk is managed and/or the hazard has been removed is related to *The Code* and your duty to be proactive in promoting patient safety (NMC, 2018b). All local policy and national guidance and legislation will change over time, so ensure that you keep yourself up to date. However, change within healthcare is a much broader subject than policy.

The future of healthcare and CPD

Changes in healthcare systems and the way that healthcare is managed have been frequently mentioned throughout this book. As a nursing associate, you need to ensure that you keep your practice up to date and in accordance with current guidance and policy. However, what drives the change in the NHS? It has been acknowledged that patients' healthcare needs and their social determinants of health have evolved over time. Patients have easier access to medical and healthcare knowledge via technology and they are living longer due to improvements in healthcare, so they have more life experience living with co-morbidities. These are the catalysts for change in healthcare, but the driving force of change comes from political and socio-economic factors. As discussed in Chapter 1, the NHS is a nationally run healthcare service funded by the UK government. Although the government does not control the NHS, they are the lawmakers who determine how much money the NHS has. Each political party in government has their own agenda and methods of achieving their ambitions, so each time that there is a change in government you will notice some changes in the NHS. These changes fluctuate throughout a government's term of office, particularly towards a general election. The availability of money is a complex process, but the strength of the economy has a large influence. Keeping up to date with changes can appear to be too much, but watching or reading the news from a source without political bias is an accessible way to monitor changes in the political and socio-economic influencing factors of the NHS.

The NHS has changed – and will always change. Keeping up to date with current changes is important, but what about future developments in healthcare that will benefit person-centred care? Considering how many changes have been made since the establishment of the NHS in 1948, imagine how many further developments there will have been by the end of this century! One of the most anticipated developments that will be available universally in the near future is personalised medicine. In Chapter 6, genomics was discussed, which is the ability for scientists to identify different genetic codes of the human genome and other organisms. This has helped to make public health more individualised because people are able to find out what long-term conditions they are more susceptible to. However, personalised medicine is completely personalised healthcare to each individual, based on their genome. Some personalised medicine is available now, and as the technology becomes more affordable, personalised medicine will become the new norm in healthcare provision. An example of personalised medicine is if a patient has pneumonia, rather than a doctor prescribing a broad-spectrum antibiotic (such as co-amoxiclav or amoxicillin) in the hope that the infection is caused by a strain of bacteria that can be treated with that antibiotic, a simple test will determine which antibiotic can be prescribed based on the genome of the bacteria or the patient. This will mean that the antibiotic will work more effectively and efficiently, removing the need to try another antibiotic if the first one does not work. There is a workforce of people already working towards making personalised medicine more accessible, called the 100,000 Genomes Project, for which there is a weblink in the useful websites section at the end of the chapter.

Personalised medicine will not be the only development in healthcare. Many technologies will enhance the capabilities of healthcare and heighten the reaches of person-centred care. Big data (vast quantities of data) will be used to predict patterns in health and could be used to mitigate the risk of epidemics or pandemics, whereas artificial intelligence (AI) will enhance the ability to manage patients' diseases, as well as the delivery of their care and their quality of life (King's Fund, 2019b). There is a misconception that technology will make healthcare professionals obsolete. However, no technology can have empathy or compassion, as technology requires programming (which cannot be done for emotions), so there will always be a need for healthcare professionals. Technology will support your ability to provide care, such as cleaning or collecting medications. This will provide you with more time to provide person-centred care. The King's Fund is a valid and reliable source of information that keeps readers up to date with developments in healthcare; you can find a weblink in the useful websites section at the end of the chapter.

Data will be an important (virtual) tool in the future, particularly personal data. You already have an obligation to maintain patients' confidentiality, as well as protecting their personal information. Protecting personal data is of the utmost importance, and the increase in healthcare technology will make data more accessible. While this has benefits for a more efficient healthcare service, protecting patients' personal information will become a primary consideration for you as a nursing associate. You may be involved in accessing, inputting, processing and sharing personal data, so you must ensure that data protection rules are adhered to. Person-centred care will be more important than ever here, as you will need to gain informed consent from patients (or their legal guardians) before sharing data. One of the effects of Brexit will be a change in data protection as the UK develops its own data protection legislation, which is another reason why it is important for you to keep up to date with political and socio-economic changes and technological advancements in order to ensure that patients are kept safe. Ethics will be an important guiding principle in determining how data is used in the future, so remember to refer back to Chapter 3 for information on healthcare ethics and law for person-centred care.

To be able to engage with and use the technology that will become more available in the future, you will need to ensure that your literacy, numeracy, digital and technology skills are kept up to date. Not only is this included in the NMC *Standards for Proficiency for Nursing Associates*, but you will need these skills to be able to use the technology, and therefore provide person-centred care. Literacy, numeracy, digital and technology skills may seem like a lower priority now, but without practice you will lose the skills you have. There are many freely available literacy and numeracy revision materials and exam questions. Consider using some of your CPD time to revise these topics, particularly medicine calculations and accurate documentation (for a suggested book on passing medicine calculation tests, see Starkings and Krause, 2018). Regarding digital and technology skills, even if you are not confident using technology at the moment, practice here will also improve your skills. Your local trust may have technological CPD training available; use this opportunity to enhance your practice, as this will equip you with the knowledge and skills you will need for providing person-centred care in the future.

Nursing associate ambassadors

'Nursing associate' is still a new profession, and one that not everyone is aware of. This requires you to be an ambassador for your profession, representing and advocating the valuable contribution that nursing associates make to the MDT and in providing person-centred care. You do not have to be centre stage on a national platform to be an ambassador for your profession. Explaining what nursing associates are, what you can do, and the contributions you make to patients and their family, friends and carers – when asked – is acting as an ambassador. Although this action may seem on a small scale, the UK government target for nursing associates in training in 2018 was approximately 5,000, and another 7,500 in 2019 (Mitchell, 2019). If every nursing associate is proactive in being an ambassador for their profession, the positive message will spread very quickly. This will not only educate people about nursing associates, but promote public confidence in the healthcare system as they learn how person-centred your care is and the service that you provide. This is another example of how nursing associates use their knowledge and leadership skills. Remember that you also lead the future of your practice.

Your future as a nursing associate is determined by you. Your focus should always be on providing person-centred care, and the content of this book will guide you in doing this. Just as the NHS will change throughout the next few years and decades, you will change too. Having a plan for what you would like to achieve is sensible and provides you with the motivation to achieve your full potential. Activity 8.4 focuses on completing a self-assessment of your strengths, weaknesses, opportunities and threats (SWOT), as well as a SMART action plan for the next one year and five years.

Activity 8.4   Reflection

This is the final activity of the book. Take this opportunity to reflect on the key learning points you have made throughout about person-centred care. It may be useful to complete a SWOT analysis identifying your strengths and weakness (areas for development) related to person-centred care, the opportunities for person-centred care development, and potential threats that may inhibit you from providing person-centred care (Sincy, 2016). Once you have done this, consider what you would like to achieve within a one-year and a five-year period.

Reflecting on what you would like to achieve within the next one year and five years is a useful way to remain focused. One year is an adequate time period to develop your practice, which may include completing a training course or moving into another area of healthcare. Five years may seem like a long period of time, but making a plan will maintain your focus on achieving your potential as a nursing associate. Your plan may change, but this is only natural as you develop as a practitioner. Remember to include SMART goals in your plans.

As this activity is based on your own reflection, there is no outline answer provided at the end of the chapter.

Chapter summary

This chapter brings *Understanding Person-Centred Care for Nursing Associates* to a conclusion. You will now have a consolidated understanding of your scope of practice and be able to identify what constitutes person-centred care. Furthermore, you are able to define the interrelation of nursing associate practice with the MDT, also known as having a professional identity. However, not everyone in the MDT – or even the patients you care for – understand nursing associates yet, so you need to become an ambassador for the nursing associate profession. This involves advocating the unique contribution that nursing associates make to person-centred care, as well as your generalist focus of healthcare: caring for patients across their lifespan and in all four fields of nursing – adult, paediatric, mental health and learning disability. Moving throughout different healthcare environments means that you will need to use your leadership and team-working skills to meet the needs of patients, wherever you care for them. As the NHS continues to change, you need to develop your practice at the same rate. Recognising the literacy, numeracy, digital and technology skills you need to fulfil your role as a nursing associate is one example of how to ensure that your practice is kept up to date. Remember that the guidance in this book signposts you to other resources. You need to use your critical thinking skills as an autonomous, independent learner as your career develops; this book supports you to do so. Lastly, as a nursing associate, always challenge yourself to enhance your practice, as well as the contributions you make to person-centred care.

Activities: Brief outline answers

Activity 8.1 Critical thinking and reflection (page 116)

The healthcare assistant acted professionally and had the confidence to be politely assertive when asked to do something outside of her scope of practice. She achieved this by remaining calm while explaining that she was not trained to change intravenous medications. Rather than abruptly refusing, the healthcare assistant acknowledged how busy the ward was and offered to do something else to support the nurse. These three actions are admirable and are an excellent demonstration of remaining within the scope of practice.

The other character in the audio recording, the nurse, could have acted differently. Rather than attempting to delegate a care intervention to a colleague who did not meet the delegation principles, she could have asked the healthcare assistant to find someone else who was competent and confident to change intravenous medication. In the meantime, the nurse could carry on with other high-priority activities and the patient in need of intravenous medication would still receive the care they needed.

Annotated further reading

Docherty, M. (2020) *What Has Covid-19 Taught Us About Supporting Workforce Mental Health and Wellbeing?* Available at: www.kingsfund.org.uk/blog/2020/06/covid-19-supporting-workforce-mental-health

This is a blog article posted on the King's Fund website. The author discusses the importance of taking care of ourselves and knowing when to seek support, but it is also a reminder to support our colleagues. We cannot care for patients if we are not caring for ourselves in the first instance. With this in mind, see Maggs (2020) below for resources that can support our mental health and wellbeing.

Ellis, P. (2019) *Evidence-Based Practice in Nursing*, 4th edition. London: SAGE.

As new care interventions, medicines and technology are introduced to the NHS to enhance person-centred care, you need to be able to engage with the supporting evidence. This book is a comprehensive overview of the research process and contains guidance on how to promote evidence-based practice.

Maggs, D. (2020) *Resources Supporting Our Mental Health and Wellbeing.* Available at: www.kingsfund.org.uk/publications/resources-supporting-mental-health-covid19

Linking with Docherty's (2020) blog article, this is a list of resources for healthcare professionals that you can use to support a positive mental health and wellbeing status. This pack of resources was put together during the Covid-19 pandemic when healthcare professionals were (and still are) on the front line of a national movement to manage the impact of Covid-19. The pandemic put additional pressure on an already high-pressured environment, so it was imperative to support the health and social care workforce. Although the pandemic is now better controlled, we need to continue to promote and protect our own mental health and wellbeing to enable us to care for patients and their family, friends and carers.

Nursing and Midwifery Council (NMC) (2018) *Standards of Proficiency for Registered Nursing Associates.* Available at: www.nmc.org.uk/standards/standards-for-nursing-associates/standards-of-proficiency-for-nursing-associates/

It is essential for you to know the NMC *Standards of Proficiency for Registered Nursing Associates* in detail. A working knowledge of the standards will guide and empower you with confidence in your practice, knowing that you are within your scope of practice at all times. Sharing this document with the MDT is a useful way to demonstrate what nursing associates can and cannot do, if anyone is unsure. The standards will be periodically updated, so make sure that you periodically check the NMC website or sign up to their newsletter.

Price, B. and Harrington, A. (2019) *Critical Thinking and Writing in Nursing,* 4th edition. London: SAGE.

Your critical thinking skills are essential for delivering evidence-based, person-centred care. This book will support you to recognise when critical thinking is needed, as well as developing your critical reflection skills and supporting you with your academic writing. The structure of this book is logical and clearly presented.

Starkings, S. and Krause, L. (2018) *Passing Calculations Tests in Nursing,* 4th edition. London: SAGE.

This book is a useful resource to help you practise medicines calculations. Although not every environment may regularly require you to administer medications, numeracy is a skill that you need to practise, otherwise you may struggle to remember how to calculate a medicine under pressure in clinical practice.

Useful websites

These are the four UK health and social care governing bodies:

- **Nursing and Midwifery Council: www.nmc.org.uk**
- **General Medical Council: www.gmc-uk.org**
- **General Dental Council: www.gdc-uk.org**
- **Health and Care Professions Council: www.hcpc-uk.org**

These weblinks will take you to the home pages of each of the UK health and social care governing bodies. On their websites, you will be able to find the scope of practice of each member of the MDT, depending on which governing body they belong to. Knowing where to find the practice standards of each MDT member, as well as your own proficiency standards, is important for knowing where the boundaries of your scope of practice are, as well as what you can ask other members of the MDT to do for patients.

Genomics England – 100,000 Genomes Project: www.genomicsengland.co.uk/about-genomics-england/the-100000-genomes-project/

Visit this web page to learn more about the 100,000 Genomes Project and the work that Genomics England is doing towards personalised medicine. This will be a significant development during this century that will improve the care available for patients, and you may be involved in providing personalised care to patients as a nursing associate. This will dramatically enhance your person-centred practice.

King's Fund – Emerging Technologies in Healthcare: www.kingsfund.org.uk/events/ emerging-technologies

This web page contains a link to the King's Fund events app, which contains information about an event that the King's Fund hosted about emerging technologies in healthcare. Lots of valuable information is presented here, so you can begin to learn more about developments in technological healthcare.

NHS Leadership Academy: www.leadershipacademy.nhs.uk

The NHS Leadership Academy has a huge number of resources about leadership and teamwork for health and social care professionals. This is a valid and reliable source of information that you can use to guide your leadership and teamwork within the MDT as a nursing associate.

Glossary

#hellomynameis A campaign established by Dr Kate Granger to remind health and social care professionals to introduce themselves, stating their name and role.

accountable Having overall responsibility for something and being required to rationalise the actions and/or decisions made.

active listening Enabling someone to tell their story without interruption and to listen with complete concentration, with an aim to fully understand the speaker's perspective.

acute condition An injury or illness that has occurred within the past six months.

agonal breathing A breathing rhythm that sounds similar to gasping, associated with a patient's end of life.

burn An injury to the skin caused by dry heat, a chemical or radiation, whereas a scald is caused by a wet heat such as boiling water or steam. There are three severity levels of burns: superficial, partial thickness and full thickness.

care after death Historically known as 'last offices', this term refers to the process of caring for a patient after they have died, as well as their family, friends and carers.

co-morbidities The physical and psychological health conditions that are caused by or associated with one physical or psychological health condition, such as prolonged stress and hypertension (high blood pressure).

communication The process of exchanging information between patients and their families, friends and carers, as well as other members of the MDT.

concordance Compliance with regulation, legislation or policy, but with complete comprehension of your responsibilities and understanding why you need to comply with the regulation, legislation or policy.

critically analyse Constructively question and debate something, examining the positive and negative aspects, to evaluate a topic, subject or event.

delegation Requesting someone to carry out a care intervention or activity on your behalf. You are accountable for that care intervention or activity, while the person you have delegated to is responsible for it.

delirium An acute condition of confusion and disorientation to time, place and person that can be caused by an infection or sepsis, hypoglycaemia, poisoning, a transient ischaemic attack (TIA, also known as a mini-stroke), or a head injury.

dementia A hypernym (umbrella term) that describes a cognitive condition which affects the function of the brain. There are many different types of dementia, the most prevalent being Alzheimer's disease.

deoxyribonucleic acid   Also known as DNA, this is the structure that contains genetic codes which determine inherited characteristics from biological parents.

dominant gene   The gene that is expressed and more active than other genes within the genome (i.e. it is more overriding).

emotional intelligence   The ability to recognise and understand your own emotions and those of other people.

end of life   Up to the last year of a patient's life.

epidemic   The high incidence of an infectious disease within a community or country.

epidemiology   A medical specialism that investigates and monitors the prevalence, incidence and transmission of diseases and long-term conditions.

evidence-based practice   Clinical or therapeutic practice that is based on the results and findings of a systematic, valid and trustworthy research study or project.

exacerbation   The process of a physical or psychological condition deterioriating and becoming worse.

gender   The social construct and feeling of being a man, woman or other.

gender reassignment   The process that someone goes through to physically change their sexual characteristics to a sex different to their birth sex.

generalisation   In qualitative research, how applicable and relevant the findings are to a defined population, environment or circumstance.

genetics   The study of biological inheritance and hereditary variation.

genome   The genetic material of an organism, including the mitochondrial and nuclear DNA.

genomics   The study of the genome.

health inequality   The disproportionate availability and distribution of health services and health and wellbeing outcomes.

health risk   The likelihood of an event taking place that is detrimental to health and wellbeing.

herd immunity   The sufficient amount of people in a population that have immunity against a contagious disease to suppress the transmission rate, usually as a result of vaccination.

hereditary   The physical or psychological characteristics inherited from previous generations.

Huntington's disease   A progressive disease of the brain that causes neurological problems such as uncontrolled movement.

hypertensive   When the systolic blood pressure (top number) is greater than 140/90 mmHg with or without medication, or greater than 150/90 mmHg with or without medication and over 80 years old.

hyperthermia   When the internal body temperature is 38 °C or higher (local policy may differ).

hypothermia   When the internal body temperature is 35 °C or lower (local policy may differ).

immunodeficiency   The inability to produce a sufficient immune response to a contagion.

incidence   The occurrence of a disease within a specific time frame.

integrity   The characteristic of being honest and upholding moral values at all times.

interpersonal   Being able to relate to and communicate effectively with other people.

lasting power of attorney   A person (or people) legally assigned to make decisions on behalf of someone else who is protected under the Mental Capacity (Amendment) Act 2019.

leadership   The action and ability to be responsible and in charge of a team with a common, unified goal.

long-term condition   An illness that has usually lasted for six months or longer.

metabolism   The biochemical processes within an organism needed to sustain life.

multidisciplinary team   A group of health and social care professionals that contribute their specialisms to meet the specific needs of a patient in their care.

myocardium   The electrical conductive muscle found in the heart.

objective   A task or activity that is a part of an overall aim.

oestrogen   A hormone, mostly found in its largest quantities in females, that causes the development and regulation of female reproductive organs and physical characteristics.

orientated   When a person understands the time and place that they are in, as well as recognising a person that they know.

osteoporosis   A disease that progressively causes bones to become more porous and brittle, commonly due to calcium deficiency or hormone imbalance.

palliative   The management of a long-term condition such as pain.

pandemic   The high incidence of an infectious disease within multiple countries.

perioperative   The care provided to a patient before, during and after surgery.

personal care after death   The physical process of caring for a patient's body, preparing them to be moved to the mortuary or funeral director, after they have died.

positive reinforcement   The provision of motivational feedback in acknowledgement of a desired behaviour or ability.

prevalence   The occurrence of diseases or health conditions in a geographical location (e.g. county, region, country).

psoriasis   A dermatological condition that causes red, dry and itchy patches on skin.

Raynaud's syndrome   A circulatory disease that causes restricted blood flow to the peripheries (particularly fingers and/or toes), induced by a cold temperature.

recessive gene   A gene in the genome that is not expressed as a characteristic due to the presence of a dominant gene, unless two recessive allele genes are present without a dominant gene.

research   The systematic investigation of a phenomenon.

responsible   The obligation to complete a care intervention or activity within your scope of practice, under the supervision of the person with accountability.

sex   In biology, the two categories of reproductive ability – male or female.

sexuality   A person's sexual orientation and/or preferred sexual feelings.

signs   Something that you observe (e.g. you may see the patient shivering).

social determinants of health   Influencing factors that determine the uniqueness of a person and their state of health and wellbeing.

stoma   In healthcare, a purposeful external opening into a hollow organ (e.g. the intestines).

stroke   An acute condition affecting the brain. There are three types: a transient ischaemic attack (TIA, also known as a mini-stroke), a haemorrhage stroke (a bleed in the brain) and an ischaemic stroke (a blockage in the brain).

subjective   Opinions or thoughts based on personal feelings and experiences.

symptoms   Something that the patient tells you they are feeling (e.g. 'I feel freezing').

systematic   A process that is evidence-based, logical and replicable.

systematic review   A research method during which research results or findings are collated and analysed from multiple studies; a systematic review is classed as secondary research, which is research of studies that have already been completed.

transgender   The personal identity of someone who has a gender identity that is different to their birth sex.

unwarranted variation   Unwanted differences in the outcomes of NHS services or processes that cannot be explained by variances in patient illnesses, conditions or preferences.

References

Age UK (2019a) *Power of Attorney*. Available at: www.ageuk.org.uk/information-advice/money-legal/legal-issues/power-of-attorney/

Age UK (2019b) *The Equality Act*. Available at: www.ageuk.org.uk/information-advice/work-learning/discrimination-rights/the-equality-act/#

Altmiller, G., Deal, B., Ebersole, N., Flexner, R., Jordan, J., Jowell, V., Norris, T., Risetter, M. Schuler, M., Szymanski, K., Vottero, B. and Walker, D. (2018) Constructive feedback teaching strategy: a multisite study of its effectiveness. *Nursing Education Perspectives*, 39(5): 291–6.

Armstrong, T. (2019) *The Human Odyssey*, 2nd edition. New York: Dover Publications.

Ashcroft, R., Dawson, A., Draper, H. and McMillian, J. (2007) *Principles of Health Care Ethics*, 2nd edition. Chichester: John Wiley & Sons.

Barry, M. (2019) Concepts and principles of mental health promotion. In M. Barry, A. Clarke, I. Peterson and R. Jenkins (eds), *Implementing Mental Health Promotion*, 2nd edition. Cham: Springer, pp3–99.

Beauchamp, T. and Childress, J. (2013) *Principles of Biomedical Ethics*, 7th edition. Oxford: Oxford University Press.

British Heart Foundation (BHF) (2018) *70 Years of the NHS*. Available at: www.bhf.org.uk/informationsupport/heart-matters-magazine/medical/nhs-at-70/nhs-at-70-timeline#2016

British Heart Foundation (BHF) (2019) *Eat Better*. Available at: www.bhf.org.uk/informationsupport/publications/healthy-eating-and-drinking/eat-better

British Thoracic Society (2017) *BTS Guideline for Oxygen Use in Adults in Healthcare and Emergency Settings*. Available at: www.brit-thoracic.org.uk/document-library/guidelines/emergency-oxygen/bts-guideline-for-oxygen-use-in-adults-in-healthcare-and-emergency-settings/

Care Quality Commission (CQC) (2018) *Nigel's Surgery: Gillick Competency and Fraser Guidelines*. Available at: www.cqc.org.uk/guidance-providers/gps/nigels-surgery-8-gillick-competency-fraser-guidelines

Central and North West London NHS Foundation Trust (2015) *Healthy Bowel Guide*. Available at: www.cnwl.nhs.uk/wp-content/uploads/Healthy_Bowel-_Patient_Information_leaflet.pdf

Citizens Advice (2020) *Living Together, Marriage and Civil Partnership*. Available at: www.citizensadvice.org.uk/family/living-together-marriage-and-civil-partnership/

Dahlgren, G. and Whitehead, W. (2006) *European Strategies for Tackling Social Inequity in Health: Levelling Up Part 2*. Available at: www.euro.who.int/en/health-topics/health-determinants/social-determinants/publications/2007/european-strategies-for-tackling-social-inequalities-in-health-2

de Bono, E. (2016) *Six Thinking Hats*. London: Penguin.

Dementia: Understand Together (2020) *Types of Dementia*. Available at: www.understandtogether.ie/about-dementia/what-is-dementia/types-of-dementia/

Department of Health and Social Care (DHSC) (2015) *The NHS Constitution*. Available at: www.gov.uk/government/publications/the-nhs-constitution-for-england

Department of Health and Social Care (DHSC) (2018) *The Department of Health and Social Care's Agencies and Partner Organisations*. Available at: www.gov.uk/government/publications/how-to-contact-department-of-health-arms-length-bodies

Docherty, M. (2020) *What Has Covid-19 Taught Us About Supporting Workforce Mental Health and Wellbeing?* Available at: www.kingsfund.org.uk/blog/2020/06/covid-19-supporting-workforce-mental-health

Edelman, C. and Kudzma, E. (2018) *Health Promotion Throughout the Lifespan*, 9th edition. St Louis, MO: Elsevier.

Ellis, P. (2019) *Evidence-Based Practice in Nursing*, 4th edition. London: SAGE.

Equality Act 2010 (c. 15) London: HMSO.

Equality and Human Rights Commission (2019a) *What Is the Equality Act?* Available at: www.equalityhumanrights.com/en/equality-act-2010/what-equality-act

Equality and Human Rights Commission (2019b) *Equality Act Guidance*. Available at: www.equalityhumanrights.com/en/advice-and-guidance/equality-act-guidance

Esterhuizen, P. (2019) *Reflective Practice in Nursing*, 4th edition. London: SAGE/Learning Matters.

Evans, D., Coutsaftiki, D. and Fathers, C. (2017) *Health Promotion and Public Health for Nursing Students*, 3rd edition. London: SAGE.

Fischer, S. (2017) Transformation leadership in nursing education: making the case. *Nursing Science Quarterly*, 30(2): 124–8.

Friel, S., Marmot, M., Bell, R., Houweling, T. and Taylor, S. (2008) *WHO Commission on Social Determinants of Health: Closing the Gap in a Generation.* Available at: www.who.int/social_determinants/thecommission/finalreport/en/

Genova, L. (2007) *Still Alice*. Bloomington, IN: iUniverse.

GOV.UK (2012) *Health and Social Care Act 2012 Fact Sheets.* Available at: www.gov.uk/government/publications/health-and-social-care-act-2012-fact-sheets

GOV.UK (2015) *Equality Act 2010: Guidance.* Available at: www.gov.uk/guidance/equality-act-2010-guidance#overview

GOV.UK (2020a) *Definition of Disability Under the Equality Act 2010.* Available at: www.gov.uk/definition-of-disability-under-equality-act-2010

GOV.UK (2020b) *Department of Health and Social Care.* Available at: www.gov.uk/government/organisations/department-of-health-and-social-care

Granger, K. (2013) *Hello My Name Is*. Available at: www.hellomynameis.org.uk

Grant, A. and Goodman, B. (2019) *Communication and Interpersonal Skills in Nursing*, 4th edition. London: SAGE.

Griffith, R. and Tengnah, C. (2020) *Law and Professional Issues in Nursing*, 5th edition. London: SAGE.

Health Careers (2020) *What Is Public Health?* Available at: www.healthcareers.nhs.uk/working-health/working-public-health/what-public-health

Health Education England (HEE) (2014) *Introducing Genomics in Healthcare*. Available at: https://youtu.be/KiQgrK3tge8

Howatson-Jones, L., Standing, M. and Roberts, S. (2015) *Patient Assessment and Care Planning in Nursing*, 2nd edition. London: SAGE.

Hubley, J. and Copeman, J. (2013) *Practice Health Promotion*, 2nd edition. Cambridge: Polity Press.

Irwin, L., Siddiqi, A. and Hertzman, C. (2007) *Early Child Development: A Powerful Equaliser*. Vancouver: Human Early Learning Partnership.

King's Fund (2016) *House of Commons Health Committee Inquiry on Public Health Post-2013: Evidence Submission.* Available at: www.kingsfund.org.uk/publications/submission-health-committee-inquiry-public-health

King's Fund (2017) *How Does the NHS in England Work?* Available at: www.kingsfund.org.uk/audio-video/how-does-nhs-in-england-work

King's Fund (2019a) *Public Health: Our Position.* Available at: www.kingsfund.org.uk/projects/positions/public-health

King's Fund (2019b) *Emerging Technologies: What Does the Future of Health Care Look Like?* Available at: www.kingsfund.org.uk/events/emerging-technologies

Maggs, D. (2020) *Resources Supporting Our Mental Health and Wellbeing.* Available at: www.kingsfund.org.uk/publications/resources-supporting-mental-health-covid19

Marie Curie (2018a) *What Are Palliative Care and End of Life Care?* Available at: www.mariecurie.org.uk/help/support/diagnosed/recent-diagnosis/palliative-care-end-of-life-care

Marie Curie (2018b) *Signs That Someone Is in Their Last Days or Hours of Life.* Available at: www.mariecurie.org.uk/professionals/palliative-care-knowledge-zone/final-days/recognising-deterioration-dying-phase

Marmot, M., Allen, J., Goldblatt, P., Boyce, T., McNeish, D., Grady, M. and Geddes, I. (2010) *Fair Society Healthy Lives: The Marmot Review.* Available at: www.instituteofhealthequity.org/resources-reports/fair-society-healthy-lives-the-marmot-review

Marmot, M., Allen, J., Boyce, T., Goldblatt, P. and Morrison, J. (2020) *Health Equity in England: The Marmot Review 10 Years On.* Available at: www.instituteofhealthequity.org/resources-reports/marmot-review-10-years-on

Maternity Action (2019) *Pregnancy Discrimination.* Available at: https://maternityaction.org.uk/advice/pregnancy-discrimination/

Mental Capacity (Amendment) Act 2019 (c. 18). London: HMSO.

Mind (2018) *Mindfulness.* Available at: www.mind.org.uk/information-support/drugs-and-treatments/mindfulness/about-mindfulness/

Mind Tools (2019a) *The Betari Box: Linking Attitudes and Behaviours.* Available at: www.mindtools.com/pages/article/newCS_82.htm

Mind Tools (2019b) *Boost Your Interpersonal Skills.* Available at: www.mindtools.com/pages/article/interpersonal-skills.htm

Mitchell, G. (2019) Q&A: everything you need to know about nursing associates. *Nursing Times,* 23 January. Available at: www.nursingtimes.net/news/nursing-associates/qa-everything-you-need-to-know-about-nursing-associates-23-01-2019/

Müller, M., Jürgens, J., Redaèlli, M., Klingberg, K., Hautz, W. and Stock, S. (2018) Impact of the communication and patient hand-off tool SBAR on patient safety: a systematic review. *BMJ Open,* 8: e022202. doi: 10.1136/bmjopen-2018-022202

National Institute for Health and Care Excellence (NICE) (2013) *Falls in Older People: Assessing Risk and Prevention.* Available at: www.nice.org.uk/guidance/cg161

National Institute for Health and Care Excellence (NICE) (2016a) *Diabetes (Type 1 and Type 2) in Children and Young People.* Available at: www.nice.org.uk/guidance/ng18

National Institute for Health and Care Excellence (NICE) (2016b) *Type 1 Diabetes in Adults.* Available at: www.nice.org.uk/guidance/ng17

National Institute for Health and Care Excellence (NICE) (2019) *Type 2 Diabetes in Adults.* Available at: www.nice.org.uk/guidance/ng28

National Society for the Prevention of Cruelty to Children (NSPCC) (2020) *Types of Abuse.* Available at: www.nspcc.org.uk/what-is-child-abuse/types-of-abuse/

Nayak, S. (2018) Time management in nursing: hour of need. *International Journal of Caring Sciences,* 11(3): 1997–2000.

NHS (2018a) *Principles and Values That Guide the NHS.* Available at: www.nhs.uk/using-the-nhs/about-the-nhs/principles-and-values/#

NHS (2018b) *Mental Capacity Act.* Available at: www.nhs.uk/conditions/social-care-and-support-guide/making-decisions-for-someone-else/mental-capacity-act/

NHS (2018c) *10-Minute Workouts.* Available at: www.nhs.uk/live-well/exercise/10-minute-workouts/

NHS Blood and Transplant (2020) *Get the Facts About Organ Donation.* Available at: www.organdonation.nhs.uk/helping-you-to-decide/about-organ-donation/get-the-facts/

NHS Design Service Manual (2018) *Design Principles*. Available at: https://service-manual.nhs.uk/design-system/design-principles

NHS Digital Service Manual (2019) *Health Literacy Content Style Guide*. Available at: https://service-manual.nhs.uk/content/health-literacy

NHS England (2015a) *MDT Development*. Available at: www.england.nhs.uk/wp-content/uploads/2015/01/mdt-dev-guid-flat-fin.pdf

NHS England (2015b) *The NHS Constitution: The NHS Belongs to Us All*. Available at: https://assets.publishing.service.gov.uk/government/uploads/system/uploads/attachment_data/file/480482/NHS_Constitution_WEB.pdf

NHS England (2016) *Leading Change, Adding Value*. Available at: www.england.nhs.uk/wp-content/uploads/2016/05/nursing-framework.pdf

NHS England (2020) *Personalised End of Life Care*. Available at: www.england.nhs.uk/eolc/personalised-care/

NHS Long Term Plan (2019) *NHS Long Term Plan*. Available at: www.longtermplan.nhs.uk

NICE Pathways (2019) *End of Life Care for People with Life-Limiting Conditions Overview*. Available at: https://pathways.nice.org.uk/pathways/end-of-life-care-for-people-with-life-limiting-conditions#content=view-index

Nicol, J. and Nyatanga, B. (2017) *Palliative and End of Life Care in Nursing*, 2nd edition. London: SAGE.

Nursing and Midwifery Council (NMC) (2018a) *Standards of Proficiency for Nursing Associates*. Available at: www.nmc.org.uk/globalassets/sitedocuments/education-standards/nursing-associates-proficiency-standards.pdf

Nursing and Midwifery Council (NMC) (2018b) *The Code: Professional Standards of Practice and Behaviour for Nurses, Midwives and Nursing Associates*. Available at: www.nmc.org.uk/globalassets/sitedocuments/nmc-publications/nmc-code.pdf

Nursing and Midwifery Council (NMC) (2019) *Our Legal Framework*. Available at: www.nmc.org.uk/about-us/governance/our-legal-framework/

Nursing and Midwifery Order 2001 (c. 1). London: HMSO.

Office for National Statistics (ONS) (2018) *Child and Infant Mortality in England and Wales: 2017*. Available at: www.ons.gov.uk/peoplepopulationandcommunity/birthsdeathsandmarriages/deaths/bulletins/childhoodinfantandperinatalmortalityinenglandandwales/2017

Prestia, A. (2017) The art of leadership diplomacy. *Nursing Management*, 48(4): 52–5.

Price, B. (2019) *Delivering Person-Centred Care in Nursing*. London: SAGE.

Price, B. and Harrington, A. (2019) *Critical Thinking and Writing in Nursing*, 4th edition. London: SAGE.

Public Health England (PHE) (2014) *Immunisations Against Infectious Disease: The Green Book*. Available at: www.gov.uk/government/collections/immunisation-against-infectious-disease-the-green-book#the-green-book

Public Health England (PHE) (2017) *Health Profile for England: 2017. Chapter 6: Social Determinants of Health*. Available at: www.gov.uk/government/publications/health-profile-for-england/chapter-6-social-determinants-of-health

Public Health England (PHE) (2018a) *Immunity and How Vaccines Work: The Green Book, Chapter 1*. Available at: www.gov.uk/government/publications/immunity-and-how-vaccines-work-the-green-book-chapter-1

Public Health England (PHE) (2018b) *Making Every Contact Count: Implementation Guide*. Available at: www.makingeverycontactcount.co.uk/national-resources/

Public Health England (PHE) (2020) *Making Every Contact Count: Evaluation Guide for MECC Programmes*. Available at: www.gov.uk/government/publications/making-every-contact-count-mecc-practical-resources/mecc-evaluation-guide-2020

Resuscitation Council UK (2015a) *The ABCDE Approach*. Available at: www.resus.org.uk/resuscitation-guidelines/abcde-approach/

Resuscitation Council UK (2015b) *Choking*. Available at: www.resus.org.uk/choking/

Roper, N., Logan, W. and Tierney, A. (2000) *The Roper-Logan-Tierney Model of Nursing.* London: Churchill Livingstone.

Royal College of Nursing (RCN) (2016) *Equality, Diversity and Rights.* Available at: https://rcni.com/hosted-content/rcn/first-steps/equality-diversity-and-rights

Royal College of Nursing (RCN) (2017) *Record Keeping: The Facts.* Available at: www.rcn.org.uk/professional-development/publications/pub-006051

Royal College of Nursing (RCN) (2019) *Nurses in Maternity Care: RCN Report.* Available at: www.rcn.org.uk/professional-development/publications/pub-007640

Royal College of Nursing (RCN) (2020a) *Legal Support.* Available at: www.rcn.org.uk/get-help/legal-help

Royal College of Nursing (RCN) (2020b) *Smoking Cessation.* Available at: www.rcn.org.uk/clinical-topics/public-health/smoking-cessation

Royal College of Nursing Institute (RCNI) (2017) *Delegation.* Available at: https://rcni.com/hosted-content/rcn/first-steps/delegation

Royal College of Physicians (RCP) (2017) *National Early Warning Score 2.* Available at: www.rcplondon.ac.uk/projects/outputs/national-early-warning-score-news-2

Royal Osteoporosis Society (2020) *Osteoporosis Treatment.* Available at: https://theros.org.uk/information-and-support/osteoporosis-treatment/

Sharma, M. (2016) *Theoretical Foundations of Health Education and Health Promotion,* 3rd edition. Burlington, MA: Jones & Bartlett.

Short, S. and Mollborn, S. (2015) Social determinants and health behaviours: conceptual frames and empirical advances. *Current Opinion in Psychology,* 5: 78–84.

Sincy, P. (2016) SWOT analysis in nursing. *International Journal of Nursing Care,* 4(1): 34–7.

Skills for Health (2019) *Resources.* Available at: www.skillsforhealth.org.uk/resources

Souza, G., Peduzzi, M., Marcelino da Silva, J. and Carvalho, B. (2016) Teamwork in nursing: restricted to nursing professionals or an interprofessional collaboration? *Journal of School Nursing,* 50(4): 640–7.

Starkings, S. and Krause, L. (2018) *Passing Calculations Tests in Nursing,* 4th edition. London: SAGE.

Suicide Act 1961 (c. 60). London: HMSO.

Tait, D., James, J., Williams, C. and Barton, D. (2016) *Acute and Critical Care in Adult Nursing,* 2nd edition. London: SAGE.

UK Parliament (2019) *How Are Laws Made?* Available at: www.parliament.uk/about/how/laws/

Williams, E., Buck, D. and Babalola, G. (2020) *What Are Health Inequalities?* Available at: www.kingsfund.org.uk/publications/what-are-health-inequalities

Williams, S. and Rutter, L. (2019) *The Practice Educator's Handbook,* 4th edition. London: SAGE.

Willis, P. (2015) *Shape of Caring Review (Raising the Bar).* Available at: www.hee.nhs.uk/our-work/shape-caring-review

Wilson, J. (2015) *Guidance for Staff Responsible for Care After Death.* Available at: http://endoflifecareambitions.org.uk/wp-content/uploads/2019/03/care-after-death-2nd-edition.pdf

Woogara, N. (2012) 10 ways to effectively manage your time on the ward. *Nursing Times,* 30 March. Available at: www.nursingtimes.net/archive/10-ways-to-effectively-manage-your-time-on-the-ward-30-03-2012/

World Health Organization (WHO) (1986) *The Ottawa Charter for Health Promotion.* Available at: www.who.int/healthpromotion/conferences/previous/ottawa/en/

World Health Organization (WHO) (2009) *Health Literacy and Health Behaviour.* Available at: www.who.int/healthpromotion/conferences/7gchp/track2/en/

World Health Organization (WHO) (2018) *Global Standards for Health Promoting in Schools.* Available at: www.who.int/publications/i/item/global-standards-for-health-promoting-schools

World Health Organization (WHO) (2019) *WHO's Cancer Pain Ladder for Adults.* Available at: www.who.int/cancer/palliative/painladder/en/

Index